OLD SCHOOL BOXING FITNESS

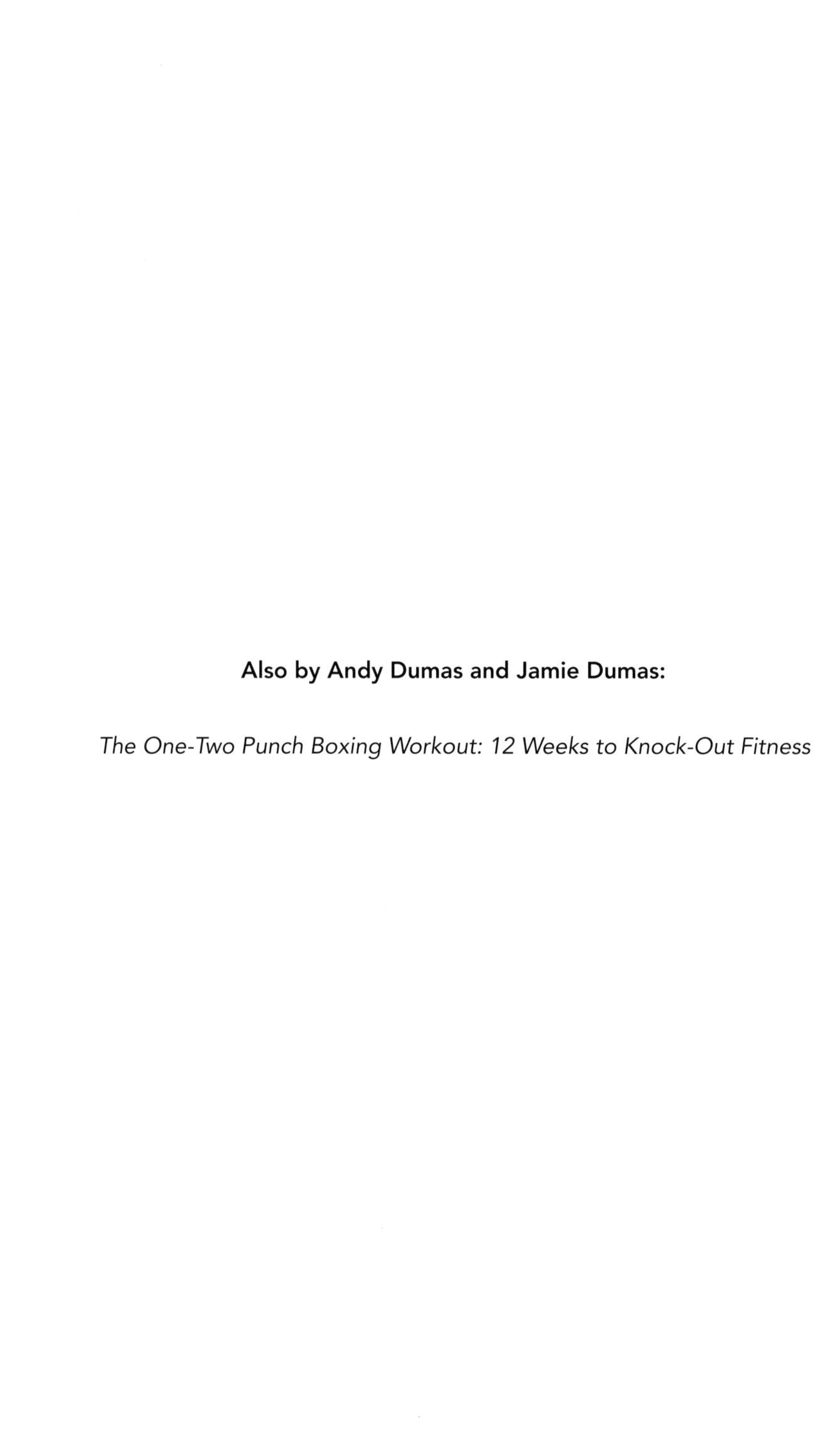

Also by Andy Dumas and Jamie Dumas:

The One-Two Punch Boxing Workout: 12 Weeks to Knock-Out Fitness

OLD SCHOOL BOXING FITNESS

How to Train Like a Champ

Andy Dumas
&
Jamie Dumas

Foreword by Julio César Chávez

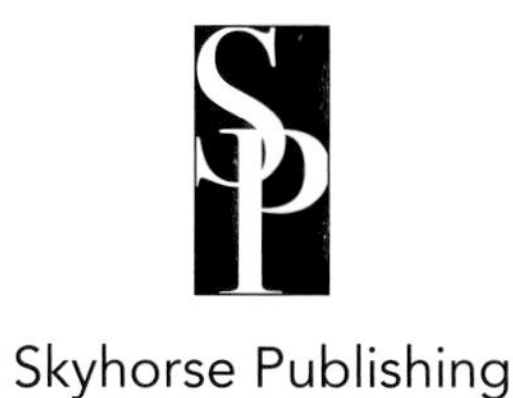

Skyhorse Publishing

Skyhorse Publishing books may be purchased in bulk at special discounts for sales promotion, corporate gifts, fund-raising, or educational purposes. Special editions can also be created to specifications. For details, contact the Special Sales Department, Skyhorse Publishing, 307 West 36th Street, 11th Floor, New York, NY 10018 or info@skyhorsepublishing.com.

Skyhorse® and Skyhorse Publishing® are registered trademarks of Skyhorse Publishing, Inc.®, a Delaware corporation.

www.skyhorsepublishing.com

10 9 8 7 6 5 4 3

Library of Congress Cataloging-in-Publication Data is available on file.
ISBN: 978-1-62087-609-1

Disclaimer

This book and the information contained herein is for education and entertainment purposes only and does not advocate or prescribe a specific exercise or nutritional plan for anyone, regardless of age, sex, or experience level.

Like all bodybuilding, exercise, fitness, health, and nutrition books, we strongly advise that you get the approval of a qualified medical/health authority before beginning any exercise program or making any dietary changes. The authors, publisher, people featured, or anyone associated with this book in any way shall not be held liable for anyone's actions either directly or indirectly.

Photo Credits

Cover photograph by **Troy Moth**, www.troymoth.com
Interior photographs by **Troy Moth**, and Ivan Krolo
Photo of *Julio Cesar Chavez* **Naoki Fukuda**, www.naopix.com
Photo of *Layli Ali* by **Naoki Fukuda**
Photo of *Muhammad Ali & Andy Dumas* by **Jeff Julian**

Printed in China

Dedicated to our Parents:

Eve and Cliff Dumas Sr.

Joyce and Joseph Lipton

CONTENTS

FOREWORD

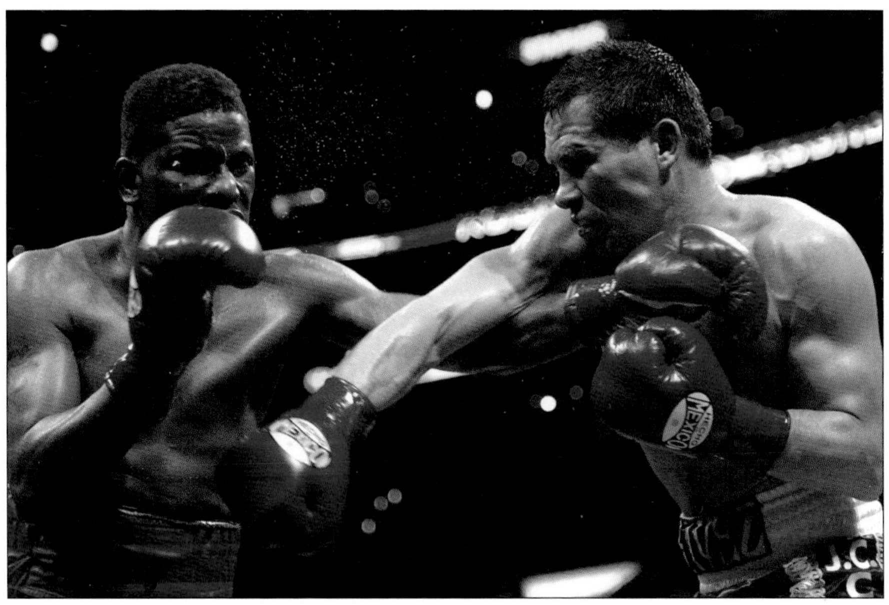

Five-time World Champion Julio Cesar Chavez

Boxing is in my blood. From my first pro fight to my final fight, my conditioning, talent, skill, and confidence allowed me to compete professionally for over 25 years, in 115 pro fights, winning 5 world titles.

Being a fighter has always been a large part of my life. I believe that pushing myself to the limit and being the best I can be has lead me to success.

Throughout my boxing career, I faced the most talented and greatest fighters in the world. Each and every time I stepped into the ring, I met the challenge with determination and the knowledge that I was physically prepared.

Boxing training works each and every aspect of physical conditioning and has kept me in shape. My muscles stay toned and strong, and my mind stays sharp and positive. The training enabled me to fight into my forties and allowed me remarkable opportunities and experiences.

At one time, the raw training regimen of boxers was only for the toughest of men. Hours and hours of training and conditioning were spent preparing for competition. Now the Old School Boxing Training Program selects the best of this "old school" training and incorporates it with the latest scientific and technical information. It gives a unique blend of old and new training routines for a complete workout for both men and women. The information in this book offers you the key to your ultimate fitness dreams, providing insight and inspiration to start and attain your own personal fitness goals.

The Old School Boxing Training Program takes you through a day-to-day workout schedule utilizing cross-training methods. The program is broken into three training sessions: boxing training, cardio-conditioning and muscle conditioning. Extensive information combined with pictures and diagrams describe all aspects of boxing training, from the basics of throwing a punch to the tried-and-true conditioning methods for cardio and muscle development.

This program offers a safe and effective path for the novice to learn the physical requirements of training like a boxer. The material is presented in such a manner as to allow the newcomer the basis for developing an improved fitness level and provides a vigorous and challenging workout for the seasoned athlete.

— Julio Cesar Chavez

Born in Culiacan, Mexico, Julio Cesar Chavez is one of greatest pound-for-pound fighters in boxing history. He won five world titles in three different divisions. WBC Super Featherweight (1984), WBA Lightweight (1997), WBC Lightweight (1988), WBC Super Lightweight (1989), IBF Junior Welterweight (1990), and WBC Super Lightweight (1994).

Chavez holds a record of 108 wins, six losses and two draws, with eighty-seven knockouts. He holds the records for most successful defenses of a world title (27) and most title fights (37). Chavez also earned the second-best winning streak (89-0) of an undefeated fighter in boxing history.

In 1993, a record crowd of 136,274 people showed up at the Estadio Azteca in Mexico to watch him knock out Greg Haugen in the fifth round. For many of his fans, this was the very pinnacle of Chavez's career.

PREFACE

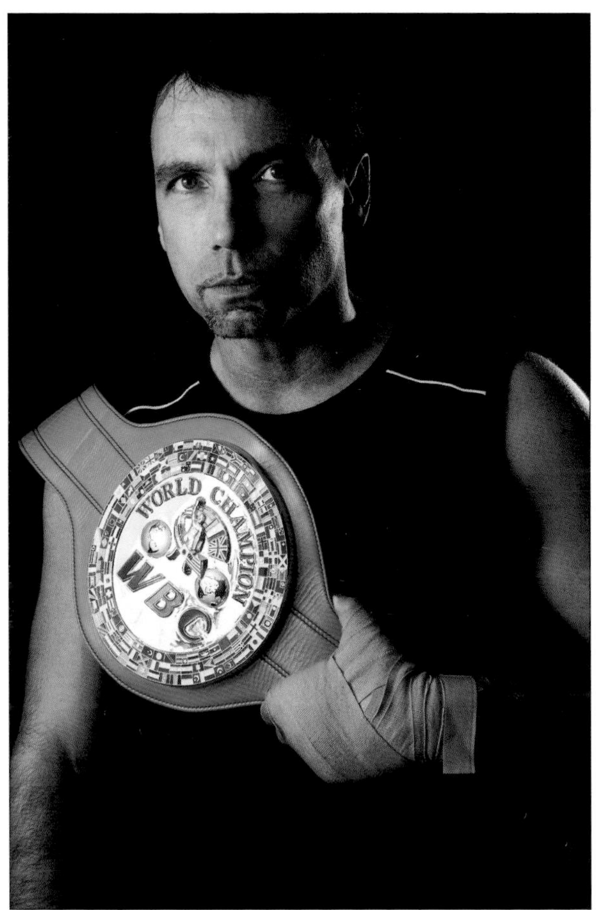

Andy's Inspiration

The fluid agility of lightweight boxers and the heart stopping power of heavy-weights can be yours without having to step into the ring. The strong, taut conditioned muscles, developed cardiovascular system, superb agility, and coordination have resulted from boxing's unique training workout. Unlike conventional workouts, boxing is not a means to an end, but an end in itself. The punching bag offers not only fitness and strength, but perhaps more importantly, sport. The agility, coordination, and spontaneous creativity required by the punching bag far exceed the mental stimulation achieved with treadmills or elliptical machines. And just knowing that you can pound the heavy bag for four or five rounds heightens your sense of security and personal confidence.

The Old School Boxing Training Program incorporates mainstream fitness with tried and true boxing training techniques and methods used by some of the world's best-conditioned athletes. With shadow boxing, target mitts, speed bag/heavy bag work, skipping, muscle conditioning and flexibility, we don't just scratch the surface of boxing in this workout!

In my early teens, I received my first heavy bag. My dad and I hooked up a chain around this great old tree in the backyard. He showed me how to wrap my hands, put on my boxing gloves, and he said one word—"Go!" Four rounds later, I was completely exhausted. I discovered that pounding the heavy bag is a great source of tension release, a primal therapy of sorts. Not only does it burn serious calories and tone muscles, it also benefits the psyche. I was hooked from that moment. This was the beginning of my passion for the "sweet science". To this day, it's still the toughest workout I've ever done.

Balance, consistency, and discipline are needed to be successful in a fitness program. These things were passed on to me by my father Clifford "Kippy" Dumas. His career as a professional boxer took him all over the United States and Canada. Originally from Windsor, Ontario, he fought in his hometown, as well as in Detroit and Chicago. He was the sparring partner to middleweight champion "The Raging Bull" Jake LaMotta, and he fought on the undercard of the last Sugar Ray Robinson–Jake LaMotta title fight.

My father had the unusual distinction of being the first professional boxer of the modern era to win two bouts on the same night! After knocking out his scheduled opponent in the first round, he was invited back for an encore match and won a decision. His passion and commitment for staying healthy and physically fit still inspires me today.

PREFACE

Over the years I've been fortunate enough to spend time with some of the greatest boxers to ever lace up the gloves: Alexis Arguello, Roberto Duran, Sugar Ray Leonard, Evander Holyfield, Lennox Lewis, Ken Norton, and Floyd Mayweather Jr., to mention a few. Earlier this year, I had the opportunity to meet and spend time with my idol Muhammad Ali. For decades, Ali has inspired millions around the world to be the best that they can be. I hope this book will motivate you to stay healthy and fit, and in some small way, inspire you to be the best that you can be.

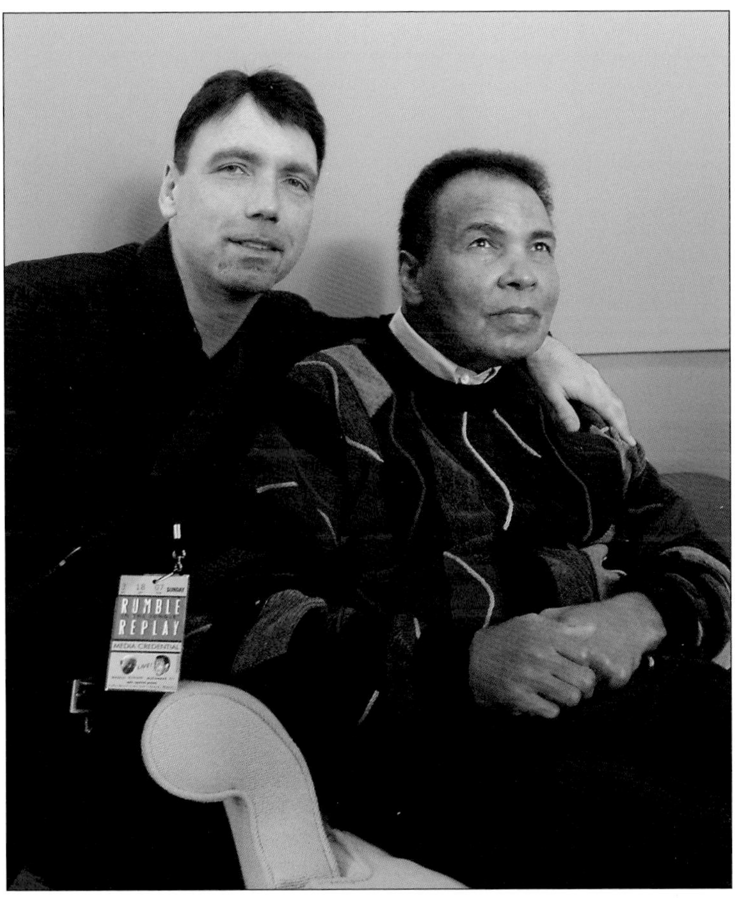

Andy Dumas with Muhammad Ali

Jamie's Inspiration

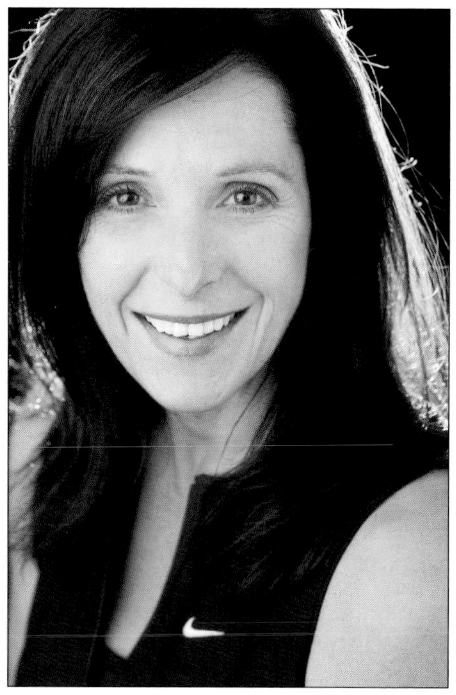

I believe in being physically active, in allowing and demanding the muscles to reach, to contract, to relax, to extend, to push, and to pull. The muscles need to be lengthened and shortened, the heart wants to pump, and the whole human body awaits the many challenges and adaptations to physical activity.

Ballet was the first physical activity I was involved in, and it includes many of the challenges a human body might ever desire. The training requires focus, concentration, a developed fitness level, commitment, and passion. The muscles, the mind, and the body must move in specified synchronism in order to produce a wondrous visual outcome. Ballet requires the development of strong, lean muscle tissue, practicing each movement, repetition after repetition, and thousands of hours of rehearsal to obtain precise timing and extreme physical conditioning.

PREFACE

Boxing and ballet are very different, and yet so similar. The commonality of practicing very sport-specific movements over and over, the focused attention, a delicacy of the reach, and the swift unobtrusive responsiveness that becomes instinctive, set these two activities aside from other sports. Both disciplines keep you in touch with physical reality, kinesthetically aware of the appendages, muscles being worked until completely fatigued, and resulting in exquisite bodies.

Take pleasure in the preparation of creating a strong, lean, and healthy body. Take pleasure in the process of the training and the development of the musculature, so that every move you request is strong and executed with perfection. Condition the heart so greater amounts of oxygen are more readily available for the working muscles, and take pleasure in the ability to create movement.

A Tradition of Sportsmanship

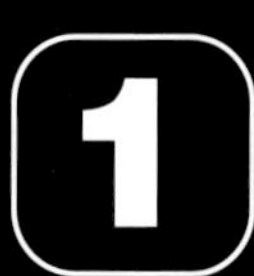

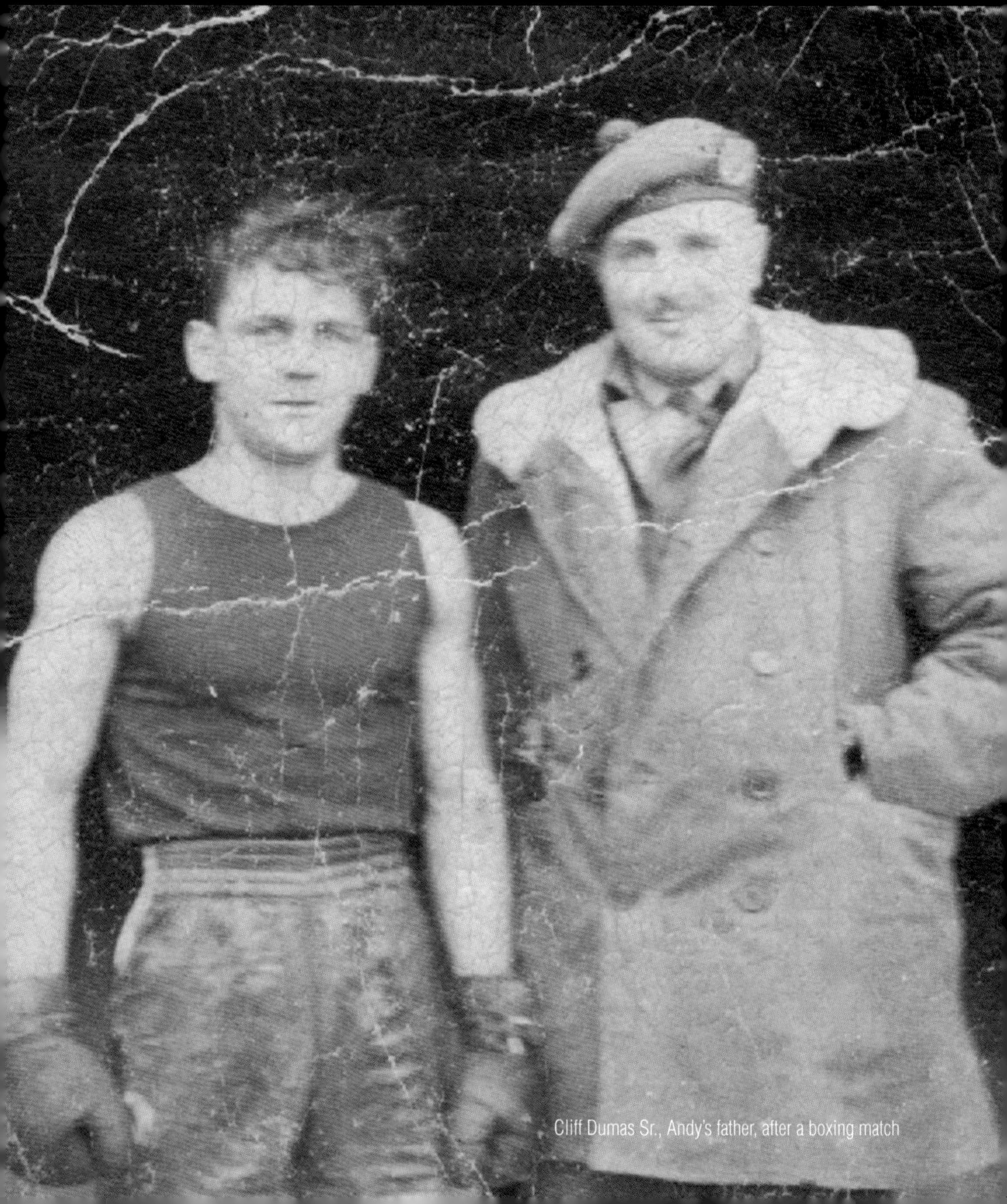

Cliff Dumas Sr., Andy's father, after a boxing match

A Short History of Boxing: "The Sweet Science"

The sport of boxing has always been a test of fitness and physical prowess. It started as a method of settling disputes that displayed a fighter's bravery, strength, courage, and brawn, and the fighter who won was held in high esteem in the community. All these elements still remain in the sport to this day, but boxing has developed into more of a contest of skill, ability, talent, and commitment. At its beginning, boxing was primal; a sport with few rules. Over the years, however, it has matured into an intricate physical science of fighting.

In ancient Greece and Rome, boxing was a gruesome sport, which combined elements of wrestling and boxing together, and permitted all sorts of dubious behavior such as biting, kicking, and the use of iron-studded thongs worn on the hands. The matches were brutal and often ended with one of the fighters seriously injured or dead. It was only when boxing was brought into the Olympics in 668 BC by the Greeks that protective gear like leather hand straps and headgear was worn during the warm-up and practice sessions. These were the prototypes for today's equipment. The Greeks recognized and prized the skill of the sport even outside the Olympic Games, and boxing took a giant step forward. Nevertheless, during the time of the Roman Empire, the gladiator style of fighting (e.g., using studded hand straps and fighting until death) became popular once again, and the appreciation of the skill behind boxing declined.

As history progressed, boxing continued to be a means of resolving disagreements in both England and Ireland. Matches in the early 1600s were held outdoors wherever an audience could gather. There were few rules, and matches would continue until one of the opponents could not get up, or even worse, was pronounced dead. It was not until the later part of the 1600s that the practice of using only the fists became the acceptable method of boxing, although punches could still be thrown anywhere on the body.

In the 1700s, gambling was part of the entertainment of the boxing matches. Town champions would be supported by financial bets and, even though gambling was illegal, the aristocracy would sponsor fighters, allowing prize fighting. Boxing matches started to move indoors and were occasionally held in the parlors of the wealthy homeowners. Boxing at this time became an elitist spectator event, creating a far different atmosphere from the old prize ring. King George I commissioned the first boxing ring in England to be built in Hyde Park, London, in 1723. Boxing was becoming a very popular pastime, and even fencing clubs encouraged members to learn the skill of boxing. The foot movements and the offensive and defensive moves of fencing worked successfully in a boxing match. Guidelines evolved and wrestling, biting, and eye gouging were no longer permitted.

British fighter James Broughton saw his opponent die at the end of their fight, and he was determined that death and brutal injury should not occur in the sport. He developed the first set of official rules for boxing. These rules, known as the Broughton Rules of 1743, were accepted by the fighters and the fighting establishments, and they remained intact for nearly 100 years. The rules protected a fighter from being continually knocked down and gave a time limit of thirty seconds for him to get up off of the ground and make it back to his side of the square for assistance from his second or cornerman. At this point, if he was badly injured, the fight would be discontinued. Previously, if the fighter made it to his feet, he could be knocked down again immediately without any time for recovery or receiving any medical attention. The new rules also stated that the fighters could not hit or grab below the waist, pull on hair or breeches, or hit a person on the ground. If a fighter kneeled, he was considered to be down, and fighting was stopped. Umpires, usually gentlemen from the spectators, were used to help make decisions on fair play. Broughton also promoted the use of boxing gloves—a lightweight muffler-during the sparring practice and introduced the counterpunch and blocking moves into the sport. Boxing gloves or hand coverings were still not used in the matches, and even as late as the 1800s, bare fists were allowed in North America. Rounds could still go any length, and it was not unusual for bouts to go as long as four hours or more. The longest fight recorded, between James Kelly and Jack Smith, lasted six hours and fifteen minutes in Australia in 1856. Fights like this one were brutal and would not be allowed today.

It was not until 1867 and the development of the Queensbury Rules that a three-minute time limit was implemented for a round with a one-minute break between rounds. A bout could go to forty-five rounds and last up to two hours and fifteen minutes. Eventually they were cut down to twenty rounds in North America, then fifteen rounds. In the late 1980s, all championship matches had a maximum of twelve rounds, and this is where it stands today.

The first state to legalize boxing was New York (1896) followed closely by Nevada (1897). Prior to this, boxing was illegal, but was tolerated at most establishments. In 1882, Madison Square Garden held its first boxing match even though it was not legal. It was not until the twentieth century that boxing became well established and legalized in a number of cities in North America and England. European countries did not legalize boxing until the 1920s and 1930s, so most fighters traveled to the United States and Canada in the 19th century. In 1904, boxing was introduced to the Modern Olympic Games in St. Louis, and female boxing was an exhibition event.

Weight classes were established in the 1850s starting with three divisions: lightweight, middleweight, and heavyweight. The actual poundage fluctuated within each class and often caused disputes in championship bouts. In 1909, the National Sporting Club determined fixed poundage for eight classes and in 1910, nine divisions were set. Today in professional boxing, there are seventeen recognized weight divisions for men and eighteen for women, whereas amateur boxing only recognizes eleven weight classes for men and thirteen for women.

Weight divisions exist in boxing ensuring competitors are evenly matched in size. It simply wouldn't be fair to have a 200-pound boxer fight a 140-pound boxer. Men's professional, women's professional, and amateur (Olympic) boxing each have their own list of classes and associated weights. The weights and classes in women's professional boxing vary only slightly from those of the men.

Professional Boxing Weight Classes

Division Name	Weight - Men	Weight - Women
Strawweight	up to 105 lbs (47.7 kg)	up to 102 lbs (46.3 kg)
Mini-Flyweight /		up to 105 lbs (47.7 kg)
Junior Flyweight	105-108 lbs (49.1 kg)	105-108 lbs (49.1 kg)
Flyweight	108-112 lbs (50 kg)	108-112 lbs (50 kg)
Super Flyweight/ Junior Bantamweight	112-115 lbs (52.3 kg)	112-115 lbs (52.3 kg)
Bantamweight	115-118 lbs (53.6 kg)	115-118 lbs (53.6 kg)
Super Bantamweight/ Junior Featherweight	118-122 lbs (55.5 kg)	118-122 lbs (55.5 kg)
Featherweight	122-126 lbs (57.3 kg)	122-126 lbs (57.3 kg)
Super Featherweight/ Junior Lightweight	126-130 lbs (59.1 kg)	126-130 lbs (59.1 kg)
Lightweight	130-135 lbs (61.4 kg)	130-135 lbs (61.4 kg)
Super Lightweight/ Junior Welterweight	135-140 lbs (63.6 kg)	135-140 lbs (63.6 kg)
Welterweight	140-147 lbs (66.8 kg)	140-147 lbs (66.8 kg)
Super Welterweight/ Junior Middleweight	147-154 lbs (70 kg)	147-154 lbs (70 kg)
Middleweight	154-160 lbs (72.7 kg)	154-160 lbs (72.7 kg)
Super Middleweight	160-168 lbs (76.4 kg)	160-168 lbs (76.4 kg)
Light Heavyweight	168-175 lbs (79 kg)	168-175 lbs (79 kg)
Cruiserweight	175-200 lbs (90 kg)	
Heavyweight	over 200 lbs (91.4 kg+)	over 175 lbs (79.5 kg+)

Amateur (Olympic) Boxing Weight Classes

Division Name	Weight - Men	Weight - Women
Pinweight		up to 101 lbs (46 kg)
Light Flyweight	up to 106 lbs (48 kg)	101-106 lbs (48 kg)
Flyweight	106-112lbs (51 kg)	106-110lbs (50 kg)
Light Bantamweight/		110-114lbs (52 kg)
Bantamweight	112-119lbs (54 kg)	114-119lbs (54 kg)
Featherweight	119-125lbs (57 kg)	119-125lbs (57 kg)
Lightweight	125-132lbs (60 kg)	125-132lbs (60 kg)
Light Welterweight	132-141lbs (64 kg)	132-138lbs (63 kg)
Welterweight	141-152lbs (69 kg)	138-145lbs (66 kg)
Light Middleweight/		145-154lbs (70 kg)
Middleweight	165-178lbs (75 kg)	154-165lbs (75 kg)
Light Heavyweigh/	165-178lbs (81 kg)	165-176lbs (80 kg)
Heavyweight	178-201lbs (91 kg)	176-189lbs (86 kg)
Super Heavyweight	201lbs and up (91 kg+)	189lbs and up (86 kg+)

Amateur and Professional Boxing

The thrill of being in command of the body, the hard physical work of withstanding the punches, practicing combinations, slipping and throwing punches, and the feel of victory are common to both amateur and professional boxing. The conditioning, the functional techniques, and the finesse are alike. The governing bodies and rules are not alike, however, and even though the outcome is the same—a winner and a loser—the fight in the ring is very different.

In England, the Amateur Boxing Association was established in 1880, and in the United States, the United States Amateur Boxing Federation (now USA Boxing), was established in 1888. Both were essential in developing the basis for clubs and for promoting safe competition for athletes of all ages and abilities.

In amateur boxing, the match is a contest of skill, not brute force or aggressive power. Fundamentals are stressed, especially defensive moves. The foundation of amateur boxing promotes an effective, fun, and safe sport, and it enforces strict rules to ensure protection. Amateur boxing requires a daily commitment to learn and develop the skills and physical conditioning. Points are awarded by landing clean and effective punches. A power punch that knocks an opponent down scores the same as an effective jab. An amateur boxer's intent is to outbox the opponent by landing clean and effective punches, rather than knocking out the opponent. The boxer with the better technique, effective punches, defensive moves, and superior conditioning will be the winner.

Amateur boxing is at the heart of all boxing and is considered the purest form. It is the essence of the sport and is highly regarded as not focusing on monetary gains. Amateur boxing is used as a vehicle to instruct sportsmanship and the values of physical conditioning. It provides a positive path to release frustrations and energies, and it builds self-confidence and character. The governing body provides certified coaching programs, arranges respected contests with bouts that are short, well supervised, and refereed: It also acknowledges outstanding athletic achievements. In 1946, the International Boxing Association (AIBA) was formed and began to govern Olympic-style amateur boxing for all countries.

Amateur boxing takes more precautions than professional boxing to ensure safety. Protective equipment is mandatory for each competition, and the gloves and headgear are required to have exact combinations of a variety of shock-absorbing foams to reduce the impact of a blow. Amateurs box for three or four two-minute rounds. The AIBA shortened the round length from three to two minutes after research confirmed most injuries occurred in the last minute of three-minute rounds.

The Olympic style of boxing is the basis of the sportsmanship of amateur boxing. Many of the great male professionals started out in the world of amateur boxing and Olympic glory, men like Muhammad Ali, Joe Frazier, George Foreman, Evander Holyfield, Sugar Ray Leonard, Lennox Lewis, Floyd

Mayweather Junior, and Oscar De La Hoya. Amateur boxing often gives the professional boxing arena its next great contestants. It is a great training field in which to learn, practice, and develop into a professional boxer.

In professional boxing, a skillful fighter is recognized and celebrated. But often fans want to see a fierce, brutal battle. No headgear is worn, and fewer safety precautions are enforced. The boxing gloves do not have the padding like amateur boxing gloves. The intent is to inflict pain and send your opponent to the canvas as fast as possible.

Rules That Have Changed the History of Boxing

Of all the professional boxing sanctioning bodies, the World Boxing Council is the leader in bringing change and reform to lead boxing to unprecedented levels of safety, fairness, and medical research for all boxers in the world.

With the creation of the WBC World Medical Advisory Board, a mandatory annual medical exam was developed for all boxers. In addition, improved medical weight-reduction systems, medical insurance, drug tests, and weigh-ins twenty-four hours before the fight were implemented.

In the 1980s, the WBC reduced championship fights from fifteen to twelve rounds. After several studies, it was apparent that the last rounds of a fifteen-round fight were the most tiring, ineffective, and dangerous. The boxers were pushed over the limits of human endurance. Muhammad Ali states that the twelve-round rule is the best rule in the history of championship boxing.

The WBC continues to research boxing equipment, the weight of gloves, and cushioning technology. Safety during a boxing match is supported with the addition of a non-scoring referee concentrating on the fighters' well-being and the application of the boxing rules. Andy and Jamie are working with the WBC to develop the World School of Boxing. The school is designed to reach all gyms of the world to help trainers and to guide them with the best procedures for physical training, medical basics, and boxing tactics through printed material and videos.

Females in Boxing

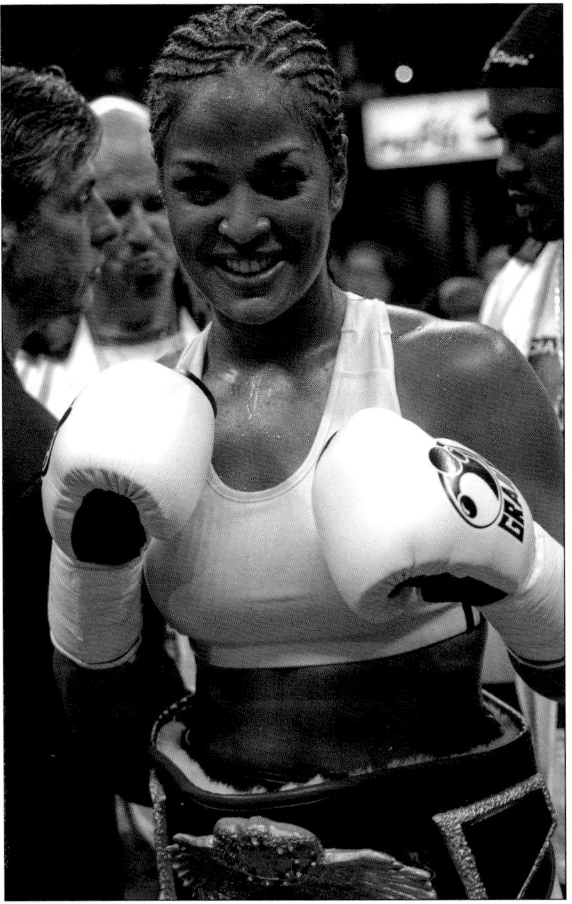

Layla Ali

The allure of boxing for women often starts with a commitment to get in the best physical condition possible. Boxing is a total physical fitness program because, as muscle mass increases and fat percent decreases, the body transforms into a strong, lean, and powerful athletic structure. The training helps to build agility, power, and endurance, as well as self-confidence and self-discipline. Boxing is a great venue for getting rid of the frustrations of the day because it combines both physical and mental demands. A boxer has to develop an inner toughness and commitment to keep going. It is the benefits of conditioning, rather than the physical contact that keeps many women involved in boxing. Boxing continually teaches something new, and because of the variety in the training, it is not boring.

Boxing is empowering and thus highly regarded as a fitness workout because making it through a session gives you a tremendous feeling of success. Women are attracted to the sport because of the skill and the thrill of incredible physical and mental discipline. Every muscle is worked. Female boxers realize that size does not matter. It is the learning and the perfecting of technique that will result in victory, and they embrace this challenge in boxing.

Women's entry into boxing has brought a new excitement to the sport, both on the amateur and professional levels. Female fights move at a fast pace with two-minute rounds instead of three-minute rounds. As interest grows in women's matches, more money is invested into the fights. Female fights are getting better coverage on Pay-Per-View events, and all-female cards are part of the entertainment scene today.

Female boxing is a phenomenon, and it was in the '70s that women really broke into boxing. There was resistance in the sport to allow women in the ring, and most female fights were considered to be nothing more than a novelty act. It was believed that women simply were not built for boxing. But, the pioneers trained hard, learned the skills, and opened up many opportunities for the female boxers of today.

The first sanctioned fight in North America, by the Canadian Amateur Boxing Association, was an amateur fight, held in Sydney, Nova Scotia, Canada in 1991, between Jenny Reid and Therese Robitaille. Canada became known as the place where women could participate in sanctioned fights. USA Boxing eventually agreed to develop a national women's amateur division. The United States joined other countries, including Canada, Finland, and Sweden in allowing women the chance to box as amateurs. There are more than 2,000 registered female boxers in the United States alone. Many people hope that one day women's boxing will be an Olympic sport, as more and more countries support women's Olympic-style boxing.

It is felt by some that it may be best for women to stay involved only in the amateur ranks, in which their skills will be acknowledged and in which there is more control of the rules. But, as the amateur base and clubs continues to grow, more women will have aspirations to experience the professional boxing world.

Jill Diamond, the chairwoman of the North American Boxing Federation (NABF) women's division and the WBC female championship committee, will tell anyone who will listen that women boxers are as committed to their craft as their male counterparts. They deserve to be recognized, she assails, and they deserve to be compensated accordingly. "The commitment of most women boxers is astounding, especially when you consider how little money they make," says Diamond. "For many of them, boxing represents something so much more than a vocation. Their devotion to the game is very inspiring to me."

The training of boxing gives a total physical conditioning, and numerous women start with this goal in mind. They attain great fitness attributes and learn the skills of the sport. They use their newly developed strength and quickness, discover the intricacies of moving around the ring, and throw punches round after round, hoping to be the first to land the punch that will make them victorious. The female boxer is articulate, dedicated, disciplined, and highly motivated. These athletes are interested in learning the sport and realizing the highest level of boxing ability and expertise.

Training and conditioning counts for the majority of time amateur and professional boxers devote to this sport. After working on fundamentals, developing the physical conditioning, agility, and style, the boxer is ready to test his or her skills in the ring and prove his or her commitment to the sport.

If You Want to Look Like an Athlete...

2

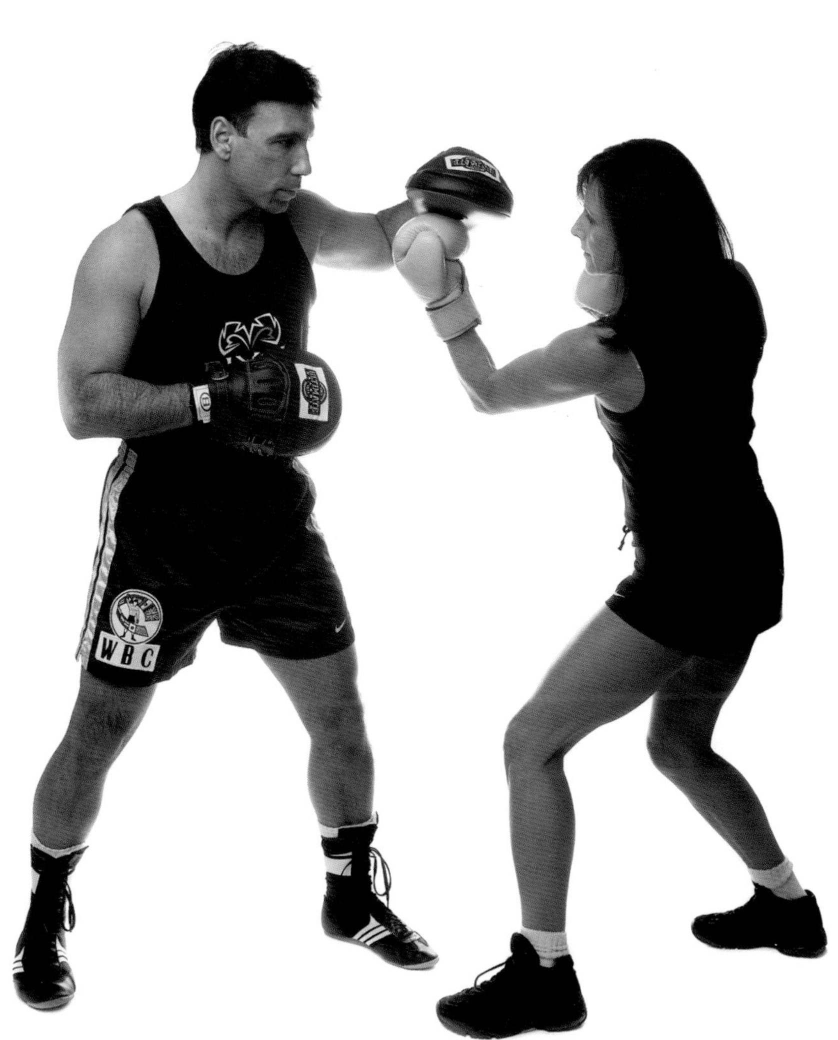

If you want to look like an athlete, you have to train like one. Boxers are some of the best-conditioned athletes in the world. Fitness boxing takes the best part of a boxer's workout and combines it with mainstream fitness, like running and weight lifting. It is a unique workout, which is not just a means to an end, but an end in itself. Anyone wanting a new and different fitness training regimen will find fitness boxing challenging and rewarding.

An increasing number of people are searching for ways to improve their physique, and many have become bored with traditional exercises. Except for those training to become world-class athletes, most people begin activities like running, cycling, and swimming with sincere intentions to improve their health and fitness levels, but they quickly lose motivation. For the average person, there is nothing inherently exciting about such exercises; they are simply routes towards the elusive hard bodies that we all crave. And without ironclad determination, it is next to impossible to maintain inspiration for something that is monotonous. The Old School Boxing Workout gives you the inspiration and guidance to achieve the best-conditioned body obtainable.

In this workout, many of the human body's physiological systems are worked, and a psychological sense of well-being is developed. The muscular skeletal system becomes stronger through weight training (muscle conditioning) and boxing training workouts. The cardiovascular and respiratory systems become more efficient during the running (cardio-conditioning) and boxing training workouts, and the central nervous system is trained to respond faster and more efficiently as it masters the intricacies of punching combinations and the execution of physical movements. Training like an athlete is hard work that leads to a wonderful sense of accomplishment and completeness.

The Old School Boxing Workout

The Old School Boxing Workout is one of the most demanding exercise routines available, and it involves all aspects of physical fitness, from the brutal anaerobic workouts to the fine-tuning of precise execution of movement. The types of activities, the placement and the variety of the workouts, and the resting and rebuilding periods will not only encourage you to continue, but will also enhance your total physical fitness level.

The week starts with the Boxer's Workout on days 1 and 4, Cardio-Conditioning (roadwork), on days 2 and 5, and Muscle Conditioning (weight lifting) on days 3 and 6. day 7 is a rest and rebuilding day. By working on all the three sessions—the Boxer's Workout, Cardio-Conditioning, and Muscle Conditioning—you can attain an overall optimum fitness level.

Some of the benefits of the Boxer's Workout include improvements in the cardiovascular and respiratory systems, increased muscular strength and improved agility, and quicker reaction times. This is accomplished by shadow boxing, working the heavy bag, practicing intricate punch combinations, heavy-bag speed sprints, target mitts, and jumping rope. This portion of the workout keeps you in touch with the sport of boxing and develops a practical skill. Learning to coordinate the muscle movements with the mind to produce a requested response is challenging and rewarding.

During the Cardio-Conditioning training session, long and short runs, sprints, and cardio equipment are utilized according to the needs and likes of the individual. It is important to build a strong stamina base, working the heart muscle to respond to higher workload demands. This base assists in future improvements in all areas of physical fitness.

The Muscle-Conditioning session develops muscular strength and muscular endurance using a variety of equipment, both free weights and machines. Training with the medicine ball offers a challenge to the musculature, and develops balance, coordination, and a strong body core.

The Old School Boxing Workout challenges the physiological systems by cross-training, reducing the chance of over-training and possible injury at any one site. The program changes from day to day, preventing boredom and ensuring positive anticipation for the next workout. The body is able to respond correctly and skillfully to the training demands because of the program design and the inclusion of cross-training methods.

Remember, training in all three areas will create a positive cross-training effect. Working on just one of the training sessions without the others does not promote the same degree of physical change or allow the body to develop into the best physical shape that can be attained. If you had to choose just one training session, however, the Boxer's Workout should be your choice. Boxing training involves muscular strength and endurance, aerobic and anaerobic conditioning. It also improves agility, response time, balance, power, and finesse.

The Old School Boxing Workout is designed for a variety of fitness abilities. Some of the principles of fitness training, adapting, overloading, cross-training, interval training, and base fitness level are reviewed.

Fitness Training Principles

Adaptation

The body meets the challenges placed on it from external sources and quickly learns the most efficient route to produce a movement. The electrical signals from the brain to the muscle tissue to produce a movement become very efficient and take the shortest and least complicated route to complete a task. The muscle responds with less hesitation and recruits fewer fibers to produce the movement. Therefore, fewer signals from the brain and fewer muscle fibers are required to produce a single movement.

When learning a specific movement for a sport, adaptation is essential in order to improve at the skill. Executing a movement over and over teaches the muscles to produce the desired outcome almost instantaneously, improving response and reaction time and efficiency. This allows for improved performance with specific reference to the skill or the sport. But when this is applied to the training of the human body and its physiological systems, adaptation enables the body to find the easiest route. The result is an efficient system that will always work at the most efficient level. The training effect—the increase in musculature, cardio-respiratory volumes, maximum exchanges of gases—will not improve unless exceedingly higher demands are placed on the systems.

The body learns quickly to adapt to the new demands placed on it, and these demands soon become old demands. The central nervous system knows how and when to execute a movement, and then the movement becomes very efficient. Form follows function, and the body and muscles always try to adapt to the demands.

The Overload Principle

One method of keeping the physiological body from adapting is to frequently change the demands placed on it. Overloading a system (e.g., running longer, harder, faster; lifting more weight more times; or spending more time on an activity) will promote and maintain an improved fitness level. But it is important not to place such an overload that the supportive and connective tissues are at a risk of injury. A gradual increase and smaller changes are safe methods of placing new demands on your body.

Essentially, when an increased workload is placed on the body, the physiological systems are placed under stress. They will try to work to meet the new demands, and in doing so, may cause some damage at the basic cellular level. The systems will require time, rest, and nutrients to rebuild, and this is accomplished in a well-designed exercise program.

Cross-Training

The workout design provides the cross-training needed for you to easily attain success. Cross-training, alternating among two or more types of activities, not only reduces the risk of injuries from overtraining in one mode, but constantly surprises the body and forces it to adjust to the diverse demands. The body performs activities, but not in the same manner as the previous workout, and the muscles and joints are given a rest and a chance to rebuild to an optimum fitness level. Training in the three different workout sessions—the Boxer's Workout, Cardio-Conditioning, and Muscle-Conditioning—results in a significant reduction in the adaptations to the exercise demands and overuse injuries. It also adds variety and fun to the program.

Interval Training

Interval training takes the workout to a higher intensity level for short periods of time interspersed throughout the training period. The overload is for a short enough time not to cause injury, but long enough to promote improved fitness levels. Workout intensities are increased gradually and for longer duration as the program progresses.

The Old School Boxing Workout utilizes interval training in the boxing training days, hitting the heavy bag and jumping rope, and in the later part of the cardio-conditioning days when sprints are performed. The increased overload lasts from twenty seconds to a few minutes depending on the type of activity and your base fitness level.

Base Level Fitness

Everyone has a starting point from which to build a stronger and healthier body. Many contributing factors such as heredity, age, and gender will influence the ability of the body to respond to the demands placed on it.

Such factors as testosterone levels will influence the ability to develop muscle tissue and to lift heavier weights. The cardiovascular and respiratory exchanges of oxygen and other relevant gases and the lung and heart sizes will influence your running ability. Fast- and slow-twitch muscle fiber percentages will influence agility, speed, and power. Limb length, muscle-belly size, tendon insertion and length, and ligament striations will also influence your initial level of fitness, the fitness level you can attain, and the sports and performance levels that you can realize.

Each individual has distinctive abilities and capacities, and the goal of optimum fitness is to try to achieve the best physical condition in the areas of muscular strength and endurance, cardiovascular and respiratory endurance, flexibility, and body composition specific to the individual. The base fitness level, the starting point or your current fitness level, will improve quickly for someone starting at a lower level than for a more athletic individual. As one becomes more physically fit, it is more challenging to attain a higher fitness level.

Fitness is such an important part of life's journey because of the health and physical gains, and the psychological, social and self-worth benefits. To begin and continue along a new and different path in life (such as daily exercise) can be exciting and motivating. But more often it is difficult to get started and to persevere.

Most have tried exercise programs, have read about them, know what they should be doing, and may even have experienced the many benefits. But just knowing what you should be doing will not give you improvements in your fitness level. You cannot just think about it; you can only improve by doing the activity.

Some of the obstacles you may face when starting an exercise program are self-doubt, lack of confidence, nervousness, and self-condemnation. These obstacles are often based on negative past experiences or times when you have not been successful in performing an activity. If you are not in the habit of training or exercising, a positive attitude about exercising will not just occur spontaneously. The emotions readily available may be only negative ones or none at all.

The mind habitually takes you back to unsuccessful times and inhibits you from performing. The lazy feeling or the feeling that you do not want to work-out occurs because the thoughts and emotions of the unsuccessful times are the ones that pop into your head. To combat this, try to reflect on moments when you were at your best. Start building successful experiences and train your mind to go to these positive times, concentrating on how great it felt and that you were successful.

If you become nervous or uneasy about performing an activity, reflect on positive experiences and stay calm. Concentrate and focus on what you are doing. Try not to give any rating to the performance, stay in the moment, and let go of the past and any failures. Remember, by starting and doing the activity, you have already succeeded. Build on this feeling of accomplishment.

Log your successes. It helps you to stay on track, and when you look at all you have done, you can draw on the experiences to keep you motivated. This is one of the purposes of the logbook and record keeping. When hitting the bag, feel the power in the arms, the contact with the bag, and the rebound off the bag. Try to become involved only in the activity, making the movements spontaneous and automatic.

Exercising regularly gives you a sense of well-being. Missing a workout day will just not feel right. On those days that you do not feel like exercising, try to discover why, and then set aside that tiny voice that keeps telling you that you really do not want to expend the energy, that you are tired, or you have more important things to do. Just start, and if it does not feel right, then stop. Most times, once you start exercising, you will want to continue. And even if you do stop, at least you had done more than if you had never started.

How we feel and perform is a function of how and what we think. The sense of well-being, relaxation, and joy carries over from the workout into the rest of your life. By making the process more important than the outcome, the outcome will result without stress and worry.

Boxing Basics

3

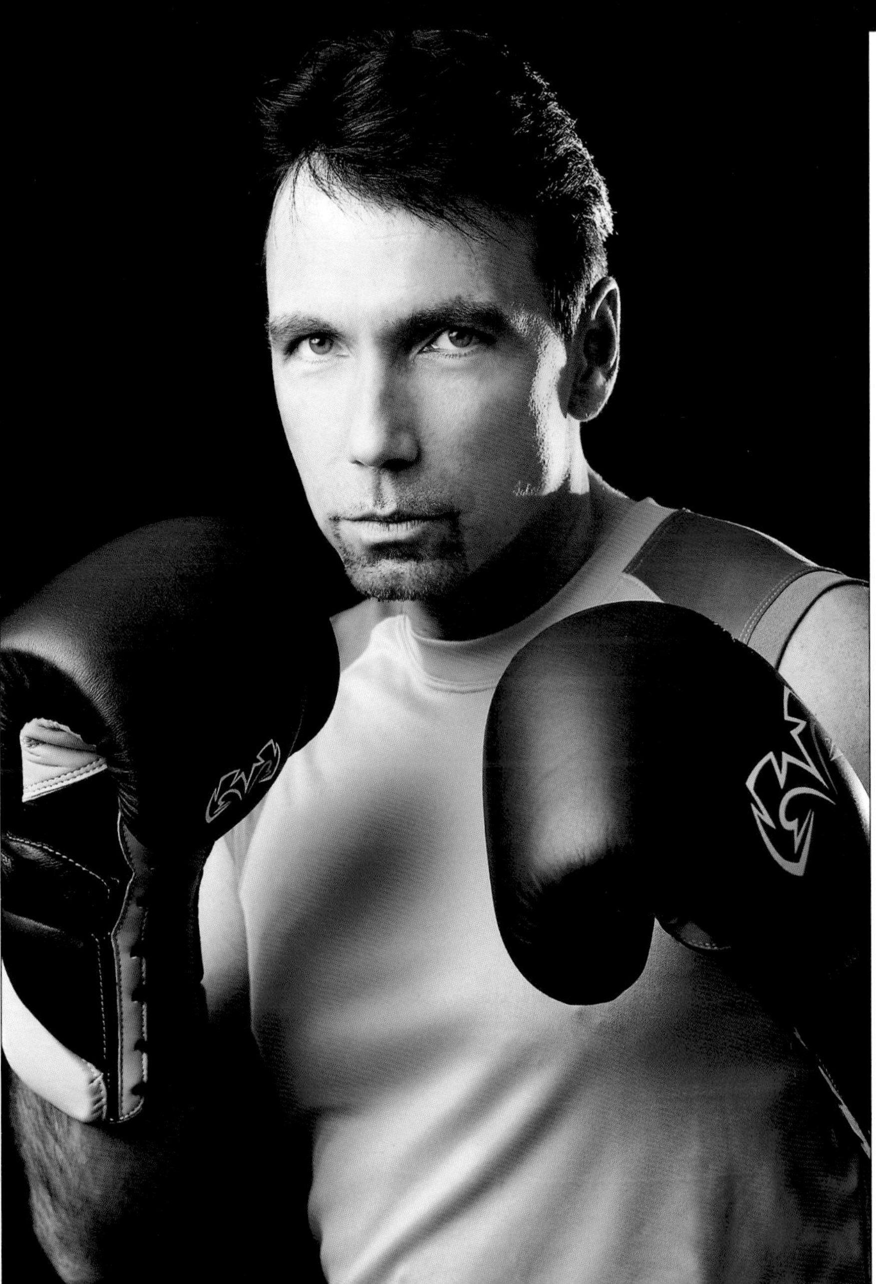

THE BASICS

Boxing stance: The classic boxing stance is the foundation on which everything is built and the starting position for all boxing moves. The classic or orthodox boxing stance is used by the majority of boxers. Stand with the feet shoulder-width apart, knees slightly bent, hips at a 45-degree angle (also called a three-quarters stance), fists up, elbows in close to the body, and the chin tucked in towards the chest. The neck and shoulders are relaxed, with the shoulders rounded slightly forward, and the abdominal muscles held tight. Keep the left shoulder pointed in the direction of your opponent and the body weight centered through the balls of the feet. Always keep your eyes on your opponent. The body needs to stay relaxed and balanced to allow a variety of movements to be effectively executed. Whether the moves are attacking (offensive) or protective (defensive), come back to the classic boxing stance.

If you are right-handed, this is the stance for you. The forward left hand keeps the opponent away, and the right arm is ready for the powerful knockout punch.

If you are left-handed, you may prefer the southpaw stance. Everything is the reversed from the classic stance. The right shoulder, foot, and hip are pointed in the direction of your opponent, and the left arm is ready for the power punches.

The Legs and Feet

Stand with your feet shoulder-width apart and the left foot forward in a three-quarter stance to the target. This is the starting foot position for a classic or orthodox boxer. The body weight should be equally centered through the balls of the feet, and the back heel should be raised slightly. The raised back heel enables you to move and respond quickly, and allows for foot rotation when throwing power punches. The position should feel balanced and allow easy movement side to side or front and back. Slightly bend the knees, so that the legs can react quickly and produce sufficient power to execute quick and balanced movements. Also, the bend at the knees will act as shock absorbers. It is important, however, not to bend the knees too much because this will cause the body to be crouched over and produce awkward and sluggish movements.

The Body

Hold the core and the abdominals in tight and the shoulders slightly rounded forward and relaxed. Focus on the center of the body, and try to make all your movements start from this area. Align the front shoulder, hip, and foot, and angle the body to the opponent, making the body less exposed.

The Arms

Hold the arms bent at the elbows, close to the sides of the body by the ribs and the hands close to the face. By keeping the elbows and arms close to the body, you are better protecting the rib cage and solar plexus.

The Hands and Fists

Hands up: Keep the fists up to protect the face and chin. The only time the hands move away from the head is when you throw a punch. Remember to bring that fist directly back to protect the head again.

Close the fingers loosely together to make a fist, with the thumb folding to the outside of the fingers. Turn the fist slightly inward. Hold the wrists straight and strong. An orthodox boxer holds the right fist slightly higher, very close to the chin, while the left fist is held just above the top of the left shoulder. It is from this position that the punches are executed. (Reverse for southpaws.) Practice keeping the fists up whenever moving, unlike the great Muhammad Ali, who danced with his arms held down at his sides. Ali had tremendous speed and agility, which gave him the ability to move away from his opponent. Fighters such as Winky Wright and Floyd Mayweather, Jr., also have uncanny ability to avoid punches from unorthodox positions. Most, however, do not.

The Head

Hold the head slightly down, with the chin tucked into the chest. Keep your eyes on your opponent and the chin protected with the right fist and left shoulder (or left fist and right shoulder for southpaws).

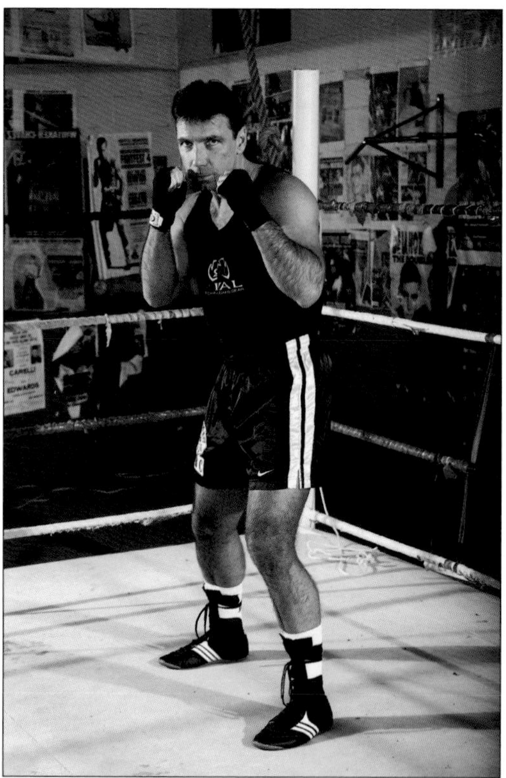

Classic Boxing Stance

Check Your Classic Boxing Stance:

- Body relaxed
- Feet in correct position, with left foot slightly forward and right foot hip-width away from and slightly behind the left
- Body weight equally centered through the balls of the feet, well balanced
- Knees slightly bent
- Torso held tight
- The front shoulder, hip, and foot aligned, and the body angled to the target

- The arms held close to the sides of the body with the elbows in tight to the rib cage
- Fingers closed in a loose fist
- Fists turned slightly in and held close to the chin

Common Mistakes and Training Tips:

The following are some common mistakes encountered by boxers. Be aware of these errors and use the training tips to correct them.

Mistake: Standing flat-footed, with the feet too close together or too far apart.
Tip: Remember to stay on the balls of the feet and have the feet about shoulder-width apart. Be ready to move.

Mistake: Shoulders raised by the ears.
Tip: Relax the neck muscles and the shoulder muscles. Lower the head slightly down towards the chest and tuck the chin in. It is difficult to keep neck muscles tensed with the head and chin down.

Mistake: Boxer stands with feet right behind each other.
Tip: A stance with the back foot straight behind the front foot compromises balance. Move the feet on an angle, shoulder-width apart. The boxer stands in a three-quarters stance to the target.

Mistake: Legs are straight.
Tip: Soften the knees by keeping them slightly bent, so the boxer can move from one position to the next quickly and efficiently.

The Execution of a Punch

When throwing a punch, the body is firm but relaxed. The legs push up, the trunk rotates, and the punching arm unwinds into an explosive, powerful punch. This synchronization among the leg, body, and arm movements develops from precise adaptation of the muscle and the continuous practice and execution of the jab, straight right, hook, and uppercut. Punching non-stop to the target, the arm travels along the same line away from the body and then back towards the body.

Proper technique is required to perform a single punch, and repetition after repetition is necessary to develop this skill. Attitude and focus also play a large part in training sessions. The mind must concentrate on every muscle fiber responding exactly in simultaneous movements. Punching imagery assists in feeling the punch, producing a stronger, better executed movement. Putting together punch combinations requires quick thinking, explosive power, overall elite physical conditioning, and many hours of training time.

The Left Jab

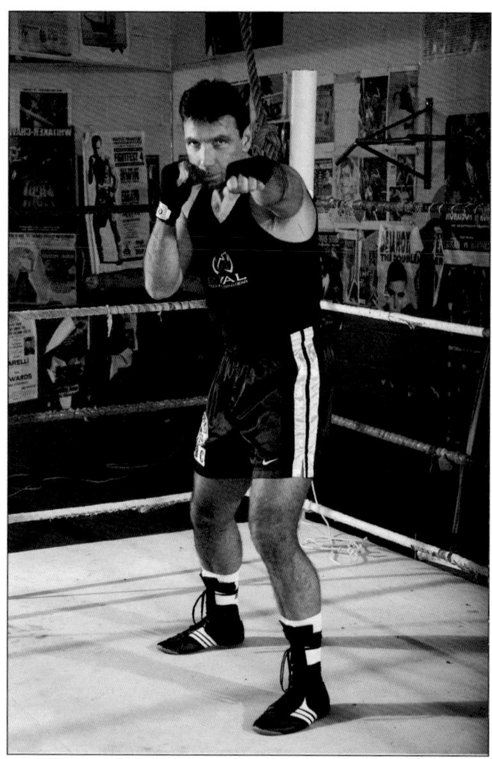

Left Jab

As the most frequently thrown punch, the main purpose of the jab is to keep your opponent off-guard and at a safe distance. It allows you to move your opponent backwards, partially obscuring his or her vision. The jab should be thrown with speed and accuracy, and you should throw it frequently; approximately seventy percent of your punches thrown should be jabs.

The jab is thrown in a straight line towards the opponent. Standing in the classic stance, it is the left arm that snaps away from the body with a slight pivot at the left hip area and shoulder. Extending this arm fully, but not hyper-extending it or "locking it out," punch the target rotating the forearm the last third of the distance. Visualize jabbing through the target. The knuckles face up and the palm down. Keep the whole body behind the punch, and push off the ball of the back foot while the front foot slides forward slightly. This all occurs just before the punch makes contact.

Always keep the right fist close to the chin, protecting it. Hold the elbow close to the sides of the body, to protect the ribs and body. After impact, bring the left arm back to the classic stance as quickly as possible, along the same line of delivery. Execute the delivery and retraction of the arm smoothly, allowing the body to remain balanced.

Vary the speed of the jab. Change the height of execution and perhaps lower it to make the opponent drop his or her hands. In doing so, you set up the target for counter punches, like the straight right. When working on the heavy bag, practice specific combinations. Try to execute two jabs back-to-back (double jab). Keep the first jab fast and light, then retract quickly, slide the foot forward, and add the second jab. Or jab to the body and then jab to the chin. Remember to execute from a centered, well-balanced position.

Common Mistakes and Training Tips:

Mistake: The fist is pulled back or drops slightly before executing the punch.
Tip: Pulling back or dropping will tip off your opponent, and the resulting punch will be sloppy and inefficient. Throw the jab from the straight on-guard position without winding up or pulling back.

Mistake: Dropping hands on the return to boxing stance.
Tip: Execute a straight-line punch away from the body and straight back to protect the chin.

Mistake: Arm does not go through the full range of motion and at the end of the punch, the arm is still bent.
Tip: A punch that ends with a bent arm will not be effective. Slow the movement down until punch range is learned. Focus on fully extending the punch and rotating the fist. Practice in front of a mirror or stand further away from the target.

The Straight Right

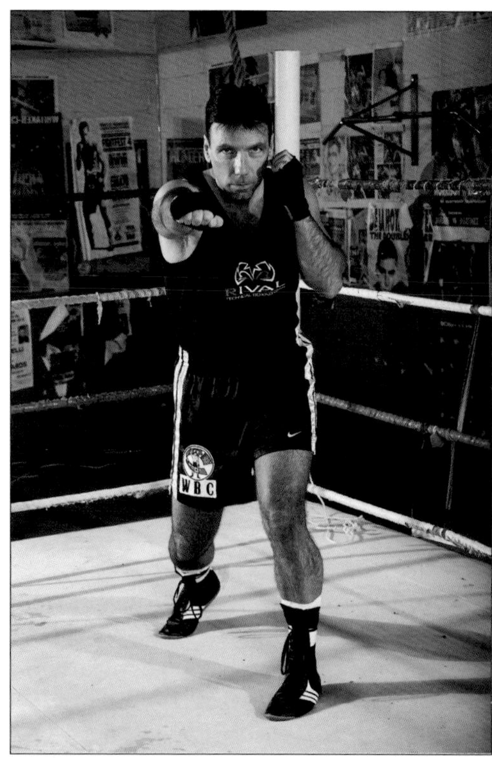

Straight Right

The power of the straight right is produced from the simultaneous rotation of the hip and shoulder, and driving off the ball of the rear foot. This punch takes more energy and time to execute than the jab. The body pushes off balance more easily, so it is important to tighten the abdominal muscles to maintain a strong center of balance and proper alignment.

Starting in the classic boxing stance, rotate the right hip and shoulder forward and extend the right arm straight away from the body. Rotate the fist the last third of the punch with the thumb going from on top to facing the mid line of the body. Be careful not to wind up, lifting the rear elbow and executing the punch in a circular motion. This will indicate to the opponent that a punch is coming (called telegraphing the punch), and he or she will either counter punch, or move out of the way. At the time of impact of the straight right, the right shoulder is closer to the opponent than the left shoulder. Finish the punch with the hips square to the target, chin down, eyes on the target, keeping the left fist up to protect the chin. The body and head are left open to counter punches and therefore, you must return to the protective, balanced boxing stance as quickly as possible.

The right cross is similar to the straight right, but with a few slight differences. It is a counterpunch thrown while slipping the opponent's left jab. The punch is thrown with a slight arc over and across the opponent's left jab, unlike the straight right which is thrown in a straight line to the target. It takes time to develop the timing of the right cross, while also keeping in mind you must stay out of the way of the oncoming jab.

Practice some combinations on the heavy bag, like the old one-two. Using both the straight punches, a left jab (one) is followed by a straight right (two). (Throw a fast left jab, then slide the foot forward to stay in range, rotate through the body, and complete a strong straight right.) Try throwing a double jab and then a straight right to the target. (Two fast left jabs, sliding the foot forward to stay in range, and then a fast straight right.)

Common Mistakes and Training Tips:

Mistake: Punch stops short of the target.
Tip: Ensure the body is rotating forward as the punch is being thrown. The hips and shoulders should move together, allowing for real power from the punch.

Mistake: The legs are straight.
Tip: This prevents easy rotation of the body and hip area, therefore minimizing the power of the punch. Emphasis slightly bent knees, thinking of the punch as a whole body movement, not just as an arm movement.

Mistake: Back foot lifts completely off the floor as the punch is thrown, reducing the power of the punch.
Tip: Practice the body movement without the punch, pressing the ball of the rear foot into the floor as the body rotates. Imagine crunching peanut shells into the floor with the ball of the foot.

Mistake: Jab fist lowers slightly just before the straight right is launched. This is an inefficient movement, which will tip off your opponent and leave your chin exposed.
Tip: Practice in front of a mirror focusing on the left fist staying high and still as the straight right is thrown. Also, touch the left glove to the side of the face as a reminder to keep the glove high.

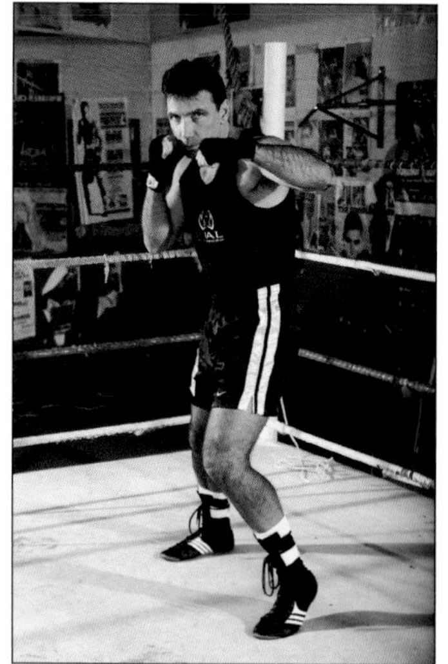

Left Hook

The Left Hook

The left hook, thrown properly, is tremendously powerful. This inside, tight punch must be executed at close range outside of your opponent's range of vision. Because of the surprise element of the punch, it is not often blocked or countered successfully. The punch is generally effective after a straight right has moved the opponent backwards [see page 45]. It can also be used as a counter punch after slipping from a straight right. The punch power comes from the force and rotation of the body, which is transferred through the hooking arm, and not from just the force of the arm itself.

Starting in the classic boxing stance, hold the torso tight and center the body weight through both legs, with the knees slightly bent. Swivel the front foot inward on the ball of the foot as you start to rotate the hips and shoulders. Pivot the entire upper body, and lift the left arm away from the side causing the under side of the arm to become parallel to the floor. Keep the elbow at a ninety-degree angle. The fist should have the thumb pointing up and the knuckles facing toward the midline of the body. The force that is created through this punch is significant and very effective, especially when it is a surprise. Finish with the elbow returning close to the body, fists by the chin and in the classic boxing stance.

In order to execute the hook effectively, throw it close to the opponent, so he or she cannot see it coming. An advantage of a left hook is the short distance it travels to reach the target. It can be a quicker and easier punch to land than the longer-traveling straight right. The hook moves about a third of the distance and is a more deceptive punch. Remember to keep the chin tucked down behind the left shoulder and the right fist held up to block any counter punches.

The left hook can be directed to the opponent's head or body. Bend the knees to move the body up and down, varying the location of where the hook lands. Practice this on the heavy bag, staying close to the bag and throwing (elbow at ninety-degree angle), on a lateral arc, across the shoulder. Set up the left hook by throwing a left jab and a straight right, (one–two) and add the hook. Spend time developing a smooth hook off of the straight right on the heavy bag, remembering to move in close to throw an effective left hook.

Common Mistakes and Training Tips:

Mistake: The arm is pulled back slightly before throwing, telegraphing the punch.

Tip: Start in the classic boxing position. As you execute the punch, simultaneously rotate the body and raise the elbow to shoulder level. Keep the punching arm at ninety degrees during the delivery o the punch. Practice in front of the mirror to perfect this movement.

Mistake: Hands drop after punch is thrown, leaving the chin exposed.
Tip: Once the fist makes contact with the target, bring the elbow down quickly in front of the body and the fists by the face to the classic boxing stance.

Mistake: The body does not rotate as a unit. This reduces the power behind the punch and throws the body off balance.
Tip: Do not push the punch, but stay loose, moving the arm and the body as one unit while pivoting on the ball of the front foot.

The Uppercut

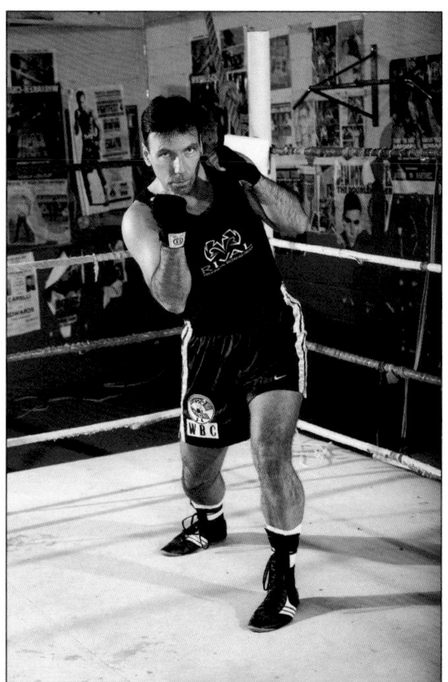

Right Uppercut

The right uppercut is a very powerful and effective inside punch when delivered to a short-range target. The uppercut is directed either high, towards the head under the chin, or low to the body, often in the solar plexus area. The uppercut can be thrown effectively with either the right hand or the left hand, with the right uppercut being slightly more powerful.

To throw a right uppercut, start in the classic boxing stance with the back (right) knee slightly bent. Lower the right shoulder to drop the right side of the body in a semi-crouch position. Remember to keep the left fist high to protect the head. Now, as you rotate the hips forward, push the ball of the back foot (the right foot) and punch the right fist up towards the target. The right shoulder will follow through with the rotation of the hips. Finish with the hips squared to the front. Always keep the right arm close to the body and moving upward in a semi-circle. For the most effective and powerful punch, keep the elbow bent at a right angle during the delivery, and follow through.

To throw a left uppercut from the classic boxing stance, start with hips squared off, left knee bent, and the left shoulder lowered. Transfer the body weight to the ball of the left foot as you deliver the punch with a bent arm at a right angle, and rotate the hips into the classic boxing stance.

Follow-up punches will depend on whether you throw a right or left uppercut, if it is high or low, and the end hip position (squared front or angled). If the right uppercut is thrown high (under the chin), this causes the opponent to straighten up and a left hook to the head is a great punch to complete this combination. A left uppercut to the head can be followed with a straight right. For both of these combinations, the body weight is shifted from side to side, and the second punch places the body into a balanced position. Uppercuts to the body cause the opponent's body to fall slightly forward. Step away and complete the combination with more uppercuts or hooks.

Remember when practicing this punch to stay close to the target. If the punch is thrown from the outside, the opponent will be able to easily detect that the punch is coming and counter with an effective straight punch. An uppercut from the outside also loses some of its power because the arm is no longer bent at the elbow and cannot effectively transfer the body's complete force in the upward movement.

Common Mistakes and Training Tips:

Mistake: Elbows held too far away from the body. This makes is difficult to execute the punch correctly, and telegraphs to the opponent that a punch is going to be thrown. There is also a greater risk of injury to the shoulder.
Tip: Be sure to keep the shoulders rounded forward and the core torso muscles held tight. This will assist the elbows staying closer to the body.

Mistake: The arm straightens out as the punch is executed upwards, making the punch less effective and less powerful.
Tip: Remember that this is a close-range punch, and the power comes from keeping the elbow bent at a right angle during the delivery and follow through. Always keep the right arm close to the body and moving upward in a semi-circle for the most effective and powerful punch.

Mistake: Standing too upright. This reduces the power behind the punch and the body is thrown off balance.
Tip: Transfer of body weight cannot be effectively accomplished when back on the heels. Get into the classic boxing stance with the back knee slightly bent, shoulders rounded, torso tight, and body weight centered through the balls of the feet.

Footwork and Movement

There is an art to moving around the ring. The boxer wants to move and shift her or his weight back and forth to set up an attack, as well avoid getting hit. Movement should be calculated and help you achieve your goal. To move effectively, you must be relaxed and in control. Always maintain your balance and stay on the balls of your feet. You want to feel as though you are gliding across the floor.

Smoothly advancing, retreating, and moving from side to side must be developed. Advancing movements are initiated by first moving the forward foot as you push off from the back foot. Retreating movements are initiated by stepping first with the rear foot and then the front foot following. To move left, move the left foot first and follow with the right; to move right, move the right foot first and follow with the left. Think in terms of pushing off instead of stepping with the foot. If you step first, the heel will strike first. You cannot move well with your heel, or change direction. The push-off, on the other hand, will keep you balanced as you can stay on the balls of your feet and move with speed and power.

Remember, never cross the feet or legs. Don't try to cover ground quickly by taking huge steps because this will throw you off balance. Work towards moving easily in any direction while staying balanced.

Common Mistakes and Training Tips:

Mistake: The feet are too far apart, causing a very unbalanced position.
Tip: The feet should always be brought back to being shoulder-width apart. Review the classic boxing stance.

Mistake: The feet and legs cross when wanting to change direction, throwing the body off balance.
Tip: Practice movement without the use of punches (keep the upper body in the boxing stance, fists up by the chin) and focus on smooth and slower foot movements. Increase the speed and direction of the movements across the floor.

Feinting and Slipping

Now that you have the basic punches and movement down, it's time to add feints and slips into the punch combinations.

Feinting is a characteristic of an advanced boxer. It requires using the eyes, hands, body, and legs to deceive the opponent and to create openings. To feint, start to throw a punch, hold back and then execute the punch. This is all done in a split second. Set up right-handed punches with a left feint and left-handed punches with a right feint. Body feints include making various movements with the body to check your opponent's reaction, such as advancing quickly, dropping your knees, or pivoting your shoulders. To set up head punches, feint punches to the body and vice versa. The opponent expects one punch and is surprised by another. Boxing is all about making your opponent think you are going to do one thing and then doing the opposite.

Common Mistakes and Training Tips:

Mistake: Dropping hands after feinting a punch. Example: If feinting a left jab, the jab hand drops slightly or stays extended too long, leaving your head exposed.
Tip: Partially throw the jab, returning the fist quickly to protect the chin.

Mistake: Making large movements and overexaggerating, eliminating the surprise factor.
Tip: Feints need to be subtle. Watch yourself in a mirror and sharpen your feints to ensure they are convincing.

Slipping is an action that competitive boxers use to avoid punches, usually utilizing a side-to-side movement of the head and shoulders. It consists of bending at the waist and knees so that the oncoming punch "slips" safely past you. The body stays directly over the legs, slightly forward and not leaning back. Return to your original stance immediately or move. To slip a jab, move the body to the right. To slip a righthand punch, move the body to the left. This method leaves both of your hands free for counterpunching and also leaves your opponent off balance. To slip hooks, move the body down by bending the knees and then lower the body under the punch.

Common Mistakes and Training Tips:

Mistake: Tipping or just bending at the waist, throwing the body off balance.

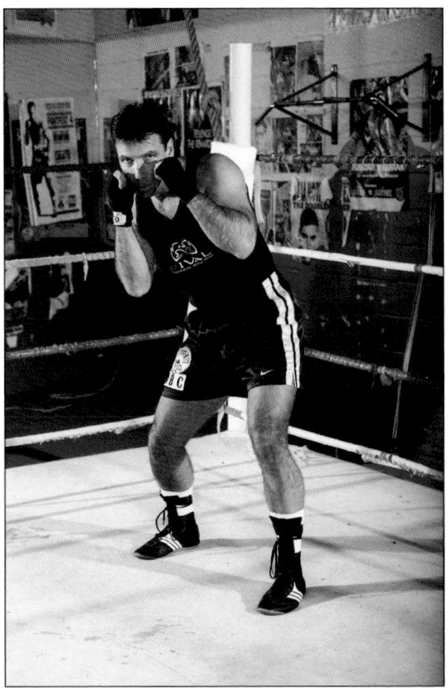

Slip to the right. When avoiding punches, don't overslip.

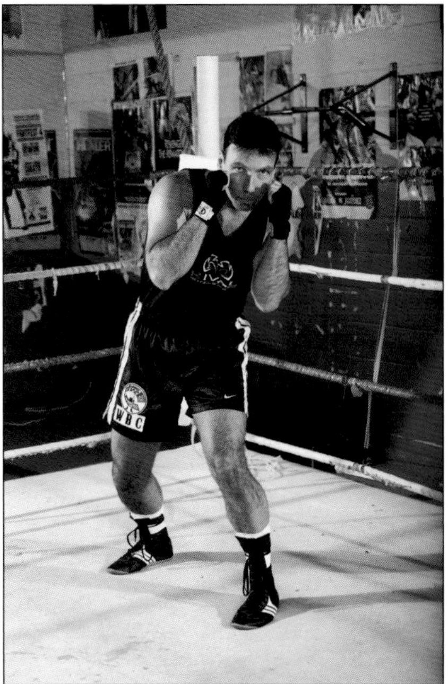

Slip to the left. Maintain balance and keep your eyes on your opponent.

Tip: Using the mirror, ensure the legs are involved on the slipping motion.

Mistake: Dropping the hands while slipping to the right or left, leaving the head unprotected and yourself unprepared to throw a punch.
Tip: Keep the hands in the on-guard position while the body is slipping to protect the head.

Mistake: Overslipping, when the boxer attempts to slip the punch and loses his or her balance, possibly falling backwards.
Tip: Practice side to side slips in front of a mirror. Establish a tight body core and a proper boxing stance. Stay on the balls of your feet and keep your eyes on the target.

Shadow Boxing

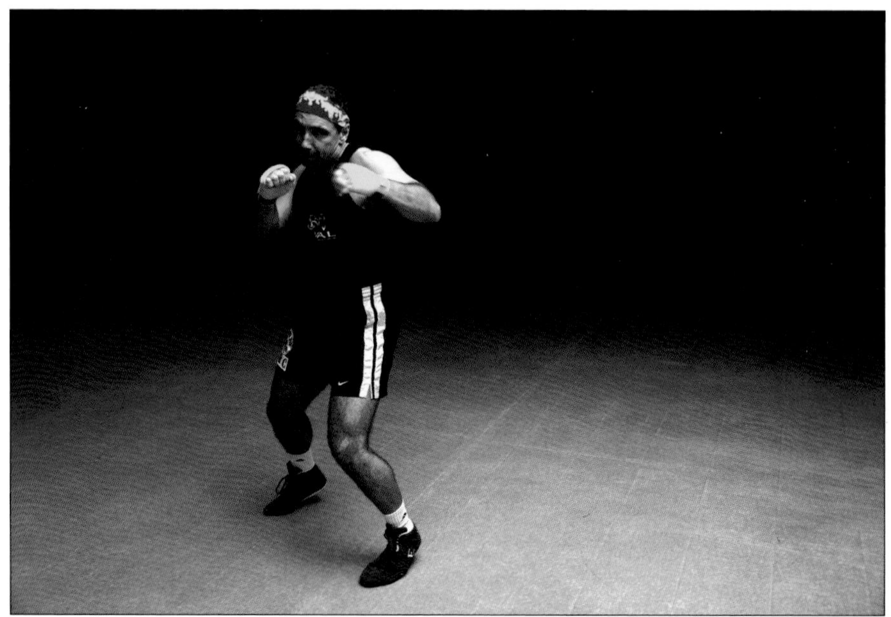

Shadow boxing. Putting the punch combinations together.

Shadow boxing incorporates all boxing techniques and is done without a bag or partner. The punches, footwork, and slipping are practiced over and over until each move leads smoothly into the next. Once you become familiar and comfortable with the actions, then it is time to start to put combinations together.

Practice moving in all four directions: forward, back, and side to side. Then, add some jabs, adding more movement and punch combinations. Ensure that the mechanics are correct and the movement feels smooth. Next, move onto the inside punches: the left hook and the uppercut. Add some movement to these punches, in the form of slips and feints. Imagine an opponent in front of you throwing punches at you, and move out of the way. Mix it up. Balance and footwork are the essential elements here. Practice the punches over and over, until one punch flows into the next. Experience the swift responsiveness that becomes second nature.

A great way to perfect the punches is to practice in front of a mirror. If a move feels awkward, break it down. You will be able to see if you are off balance, if you are shifting your weight incorrectly, if the arms are held at the incorrect angle, or if the hands are held too high or too low. It is easier to correct a punch in front of the mirror where you can see it than to wait until you are on the heavy bag. Always start slowly with the basic punches and as you become more secure with the feel of movements, add speed and combinations. If a combination does not feel right, slow it down and break it into smaller combinations until the punches and movements flow one to the other.

You should always have a purpose when you shadow box. Match the footwork with the punches, having a mental image of what you want to achieve. Keep it simple at first, then decide where you want to hit and what punch you want to throw. Try to find a comfortable rhythm and move around. Mirror training will assist you in executing the punches correctly. And shadow boxing is a great way to warm up the body by increasing blood flow to the muscles and lubricating the joints.

Shadow box for three minutes and try to recognize the length of a round. In the Old School Training program, the three-minute round is used throughout, and you will learn to pace yourself. Work hard enough so that you will feel slightly out of breath, and be ready and eager for more. Take the minute in between rounds to think about new combinations, both offensive and defensive.

Common Mistakes and Training Tips:

Mistake: Standing in one place while throwing punches.
Tip: Start moving without the punches, focusing on foot and leg movements. Add slips and feints, then jabs and straight rights.

Mistake: Dropping the hands away from the chin, leaving your head exposed.

Tip: The rule is "one hand out, one hand back." When the left hand is punching, the right is back, and vice versa.

Throwing Effective Combinations

The finish of one punch should set you up for the start of the next one. If the first punch puts you off balance slightly, the next punch should put you back on balance. For example, throwing a straight right will leave the body in the perfect starting position to throw a left hook. The completion of the left hook will bring the body back to the classic boxing stance and into position for the next punch.

Establish your punching form first. Punching speed and power comes later. It is especially important for beginners to ensure that proper punch execution is being practiced, even if it means slowing down and throwing fewer punches.

Double up on your punches. Throw two jabs or two hooks consecutively. This will throw the opponent off because it will be unexpected after only single punches have been thrown. Be aware, however, that the time between the punches will be longer because you must go back to the starting position in order to execute the punch correctly. With practice, the time between punches will decrease as the body learns to move in and out of position quickly.

Try to vary the height of the punches. Not only will this give you a better overall workout, it will also keep the opponent on guard. Practice throwing punches to the body area, then throw a few higher-placed punches. Incorporate feints and slips, moving the body from side to side. Also vary the speed of the punches. Do not to be predictable! For example, throw a left jab at three-quarter speed and then one really strong fast jab.

Classic Combinations

Double and Triple Jabs

- The one-two (this is a left jab followed by a straight right.)

- One–two–hook (Left jab, straight right, left hook)
- Right uppercut–left hook
- Left jab–left hook–straight right–left hook
- Left jab–left hook to the body–left hook to the head–straight right
- Left jab–left uppercut to the body–left hook to the chin
- Left uppercut to the body–straight right to the head
- Left jab to the body–left jab to the head
- One–two to the body–one–two to the head (left jab, straight right to the body, left jab, straight right to the body)

Think about the punches and learn which one is your most effective and preferred. Place your best or favorite punch at the end of a sequence. Mix it up! Order the punches so that you will finish in balance and in the classic boxing stance, ready to move quickly into the next move.

Working the Bags

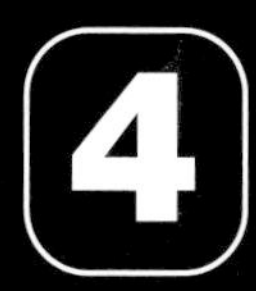

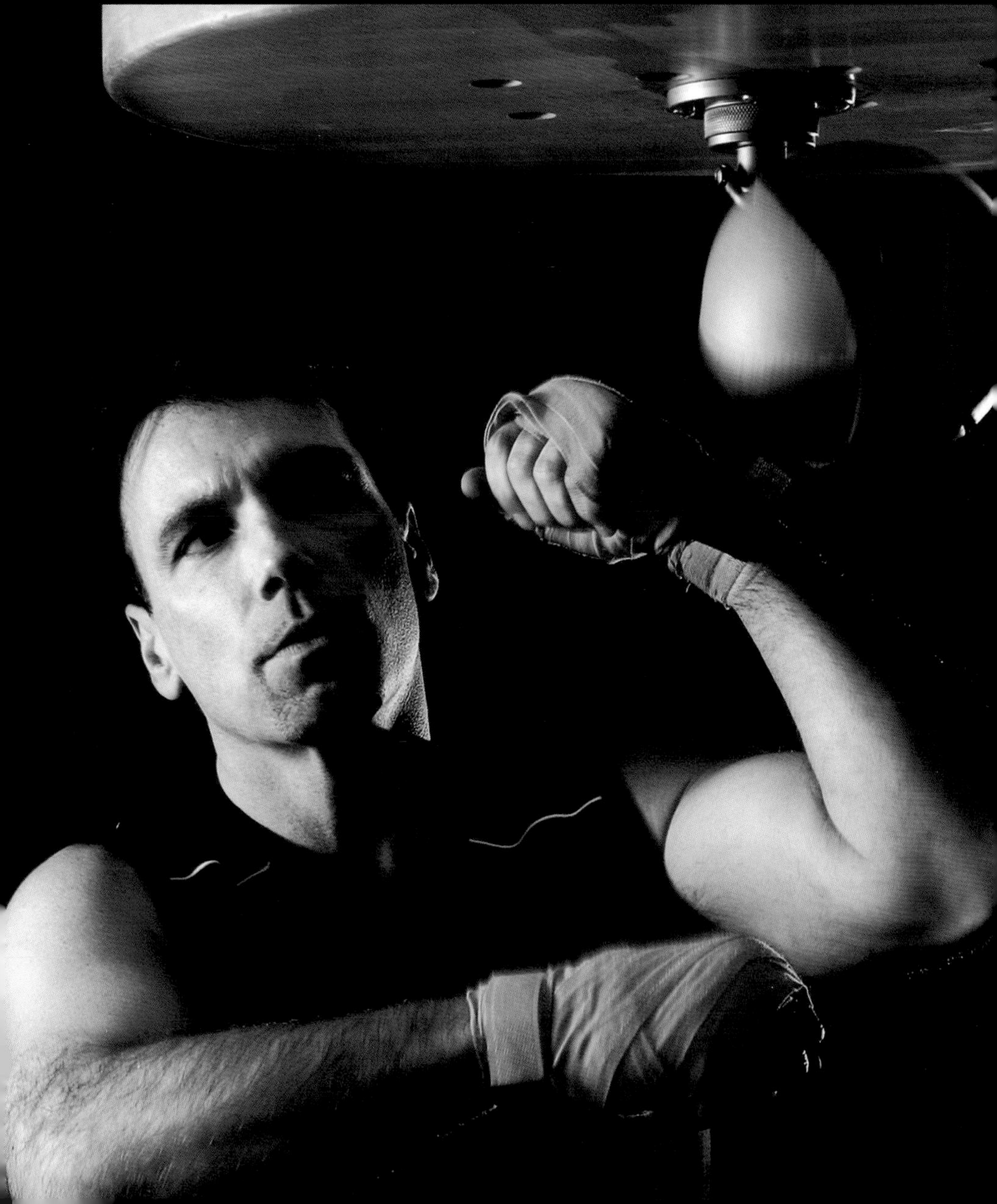

Working the Bags

Training on the heavy bag, speed bag, and double-end bag provides instantaneous feedback and teaches you about your technique, ability, and punching style. Directing the punches to the heavy bag is a great release of tension, builds punching power and strength, and also gives you the chance to feel the power, strength, and speed behind your punches. Hitting the speed bag develops quickness and improves coordination. Punching the double-end bag tests and develops your agility and reaction time.

Before you put on the gloves and start the workout of your life, it is important to protect your hands with wraps.

Protecting Your Hands

Hand Wraps

Reusable protective bandages are wrapped around the wrists, hands, and knuckles to give wrist support, protect the small bones, and prevent abrasions of the knuckles. The wrists and hands become one strong unit, which

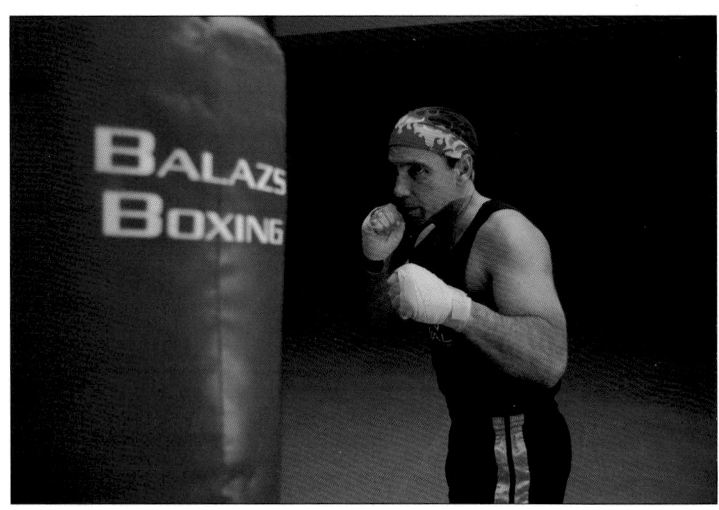

is important when hitting the heavy bag. There are a number of different techniques of hand wrapping, and each is ritualistic to the coach and boxer. It is important to wrap with an even tension and not too tight at any one place. The wrap should feel snug enough to give support, but not so tight that the circulation is impinged. Wrapping the same way each time will help you determine the right amount of tension. It needs to be noted that there are numerous styles and lengths of hand wraps. For the hand-wrapping technique below, a 160- to 180-inch wrap is required to give support to the wrists and protect the hands.

How to Wrap your Hands:

Step 1: Place the loop of the wrap around the thumb, with the wrap falling to the front side of the wrist. Keep the hand open and relaxed, with your fingers spread open.
Step 2: Wrap twice around the wrist and then once around the thumb.
Step 3: Spread your fingers and wrap around the knuckles four to five times. Keeping the wrap flat, without any bulges, overlap the side edges slightly to prevent spaces where the skin could extend through.
Step 4: Take the wrap under the palm up to the wrist, and bring it across the back of the hand between the small and ring finger. Repeat bringing the wrap under the palm and up over the back of the hand between the ring finger and the long finger. Continue with the last finger up to the wrist.
Step 5: From the wrist, wrap around the knuckles two to three times.
Step 6: With the remainder, continue to wrap around the wrist and hand in a figure-eight pattern.
Step 7: Leave enough wrap to finish two to three times around the wrist, and secure the Velcro fasteners or ties.

Hand wraps should always be worn under your gloves. They can be used on their own when working on the speed bag or when practicing light punching technique on the double-end bag. Otherwise, either a boxing glove or a striking mitt covers them.

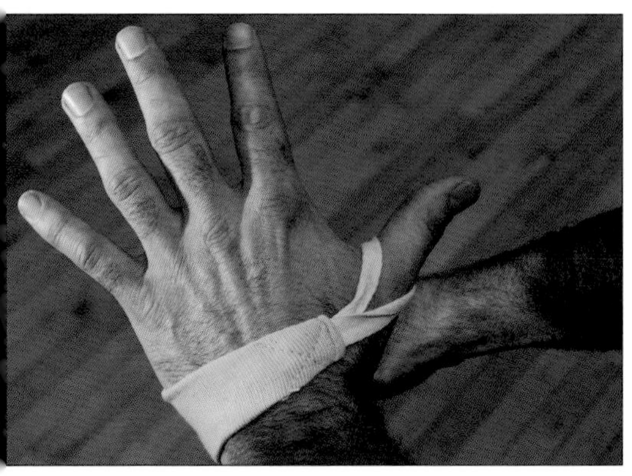

The loop of the wrap is placed around the thumb.

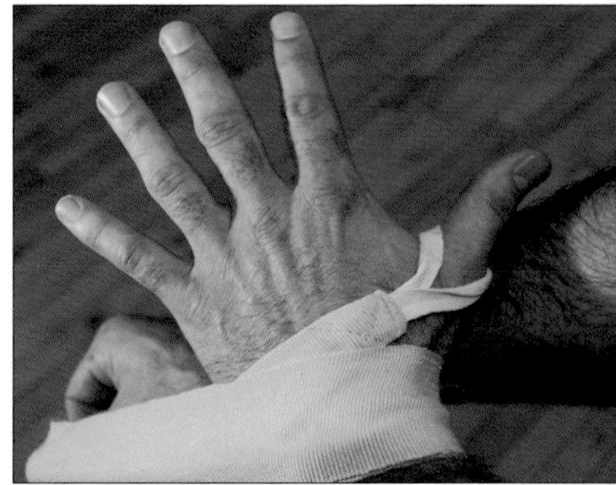

Wrap twice around the wrist.

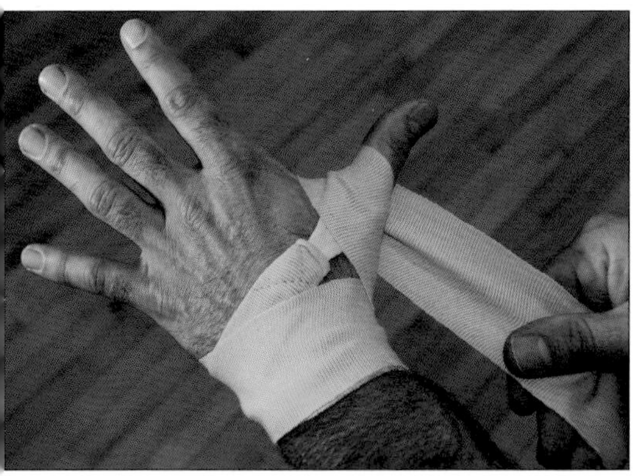

Wrap around the thumb.

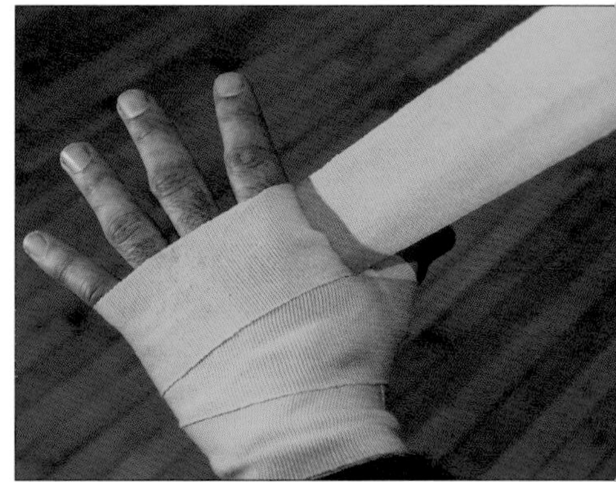

Wrap around the knuckles four to five times.

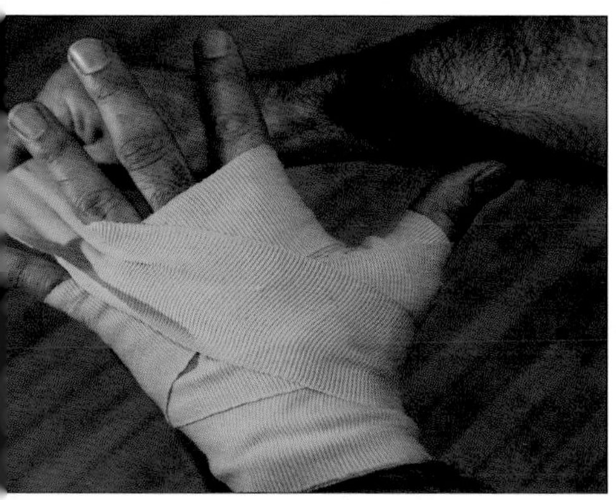
Wrap between the little finger and ring finger.

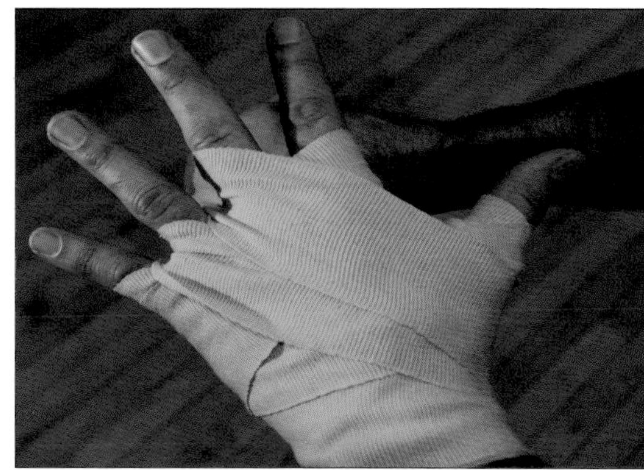
Wrap between the ring finger and long finger.

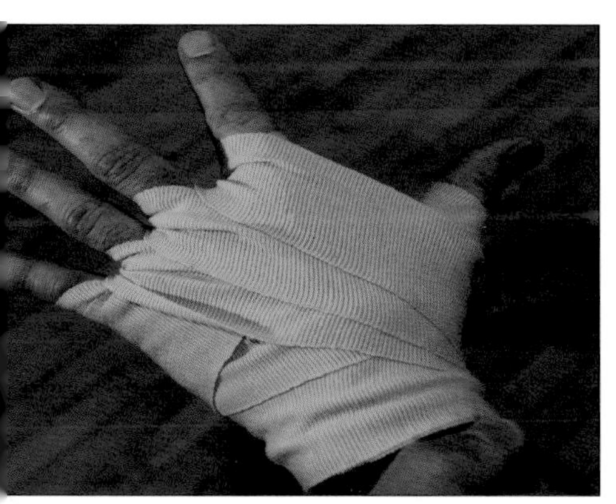
Wrap between the long finger and last finger.

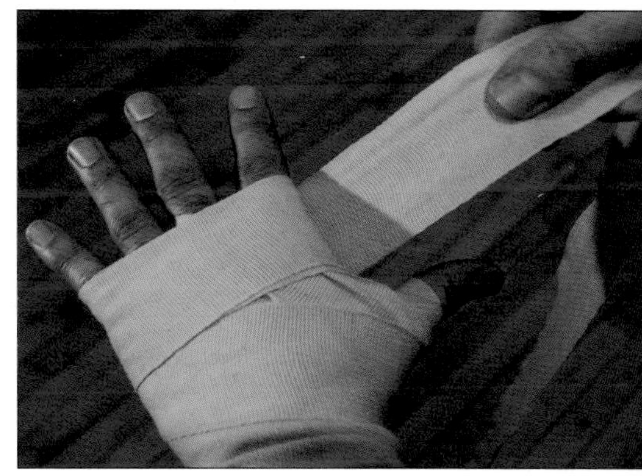
Wrap around the knuckles two to three times.

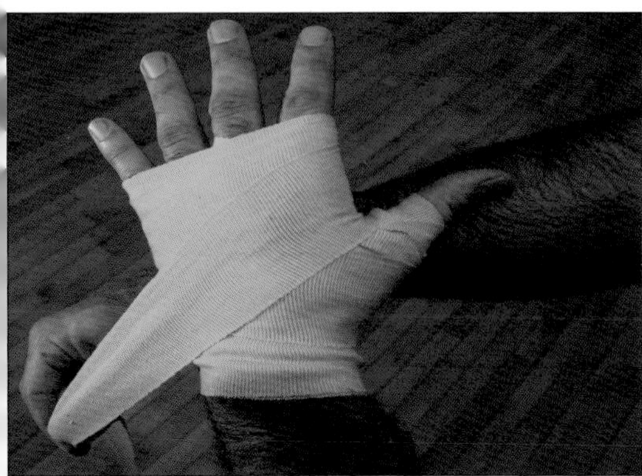

Wrap once around the wrist.

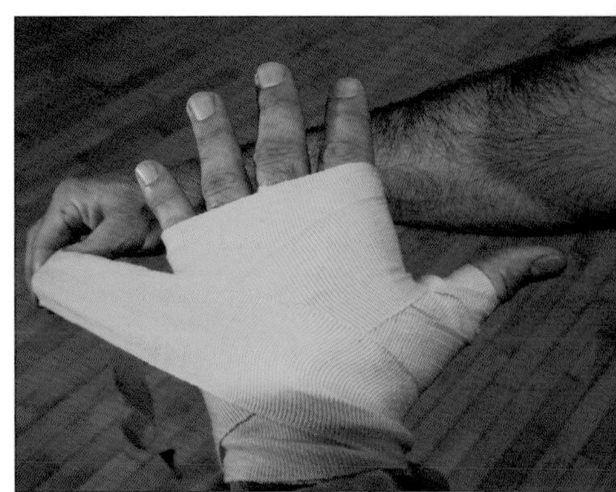

And once around the hand in a figure eight for a few times.

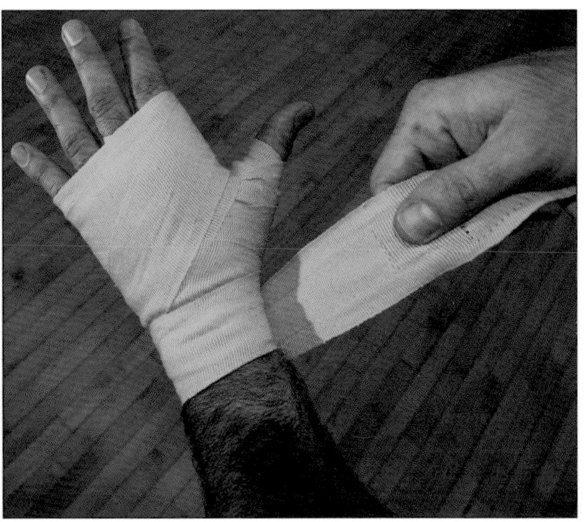

Around the wrist two to three times.

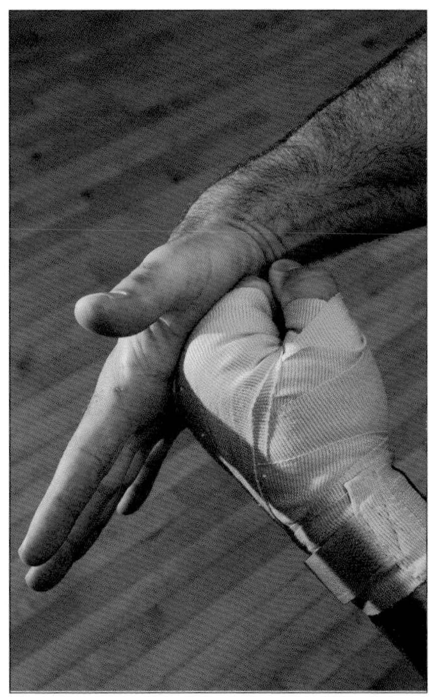

Secure to finish.

Types of Gloves

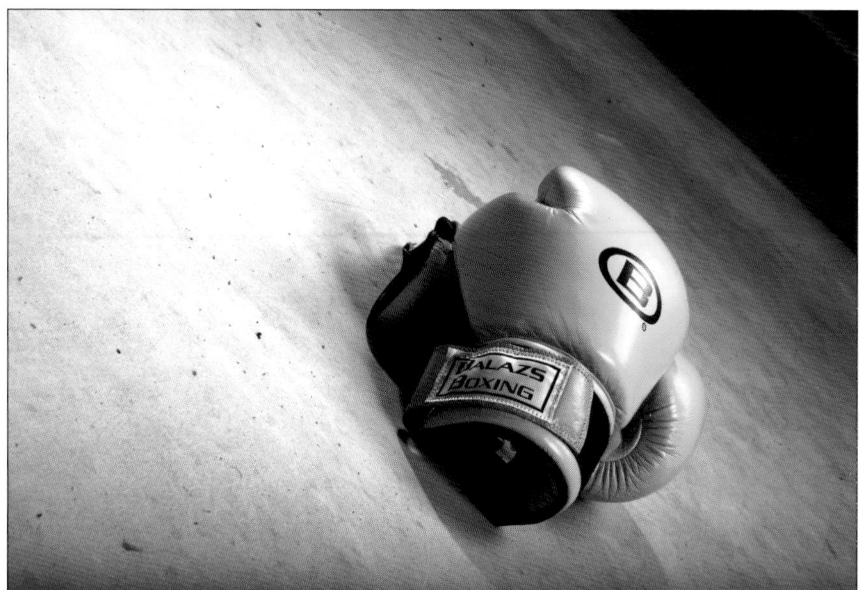

Heavy Bag Gloves

Heavy bag gloves are worn during training sessions on the bags and on the target mitts. They give additional protection to the hands and wrists, especially when pounding the heavy bag—and they protect the knuckles with the extra padding inside. The gloves require sufficient room inside to allow for circulation in the hand, but they should not be so roomy that the hand moves around. The palms of the some makes of gloves are slightly padded and molded to ensure a secure fit around the hand. Heavy bag gloves have Velcro fasteners, which give the wrist great support and make it easy to put on and off. The exterior of the gloves is made of leather and the interior of foam padding. Personal preference will dictate the weight of the glove you choose, anywhere from ten to sixteen ounces. It is important for the gloves to feel comfortable and have adequate padding to absorb the shock of the impact on the heavy bag.

Sparring Gloves

Sparring gloves are designed differently from bag gloves because they are used to strike an opponent rather than a heavy bag. They have extra shock absorbing foam and should be anywhere from fourteen to twenty ounces. A thumb strap is found on sparring and boxing gloves today. This protects the thumb from being sprained or dislocated and protects the opponent from getting a thumb in the eye.

Boxing Gloves

Boxing gloves used in matches generally weigh eight or ten ounces. They have laces to fasten them at the wrist area and then are taped around the wrist for additional wrist support and prevention of the glove becoming loose.

Gloves should be used specifically what they are designed for. Bag gloves should not be used for sparring, and sparring gloves should not be used on the heavy bag.

Working the Bags

The Heavy Bag

There are a variety of materials, sizes, and weights of heavy bags specific to training needs and individual requirements. The materials used on the bags range from leather—the most durable and expensive—to canvas, which is the least expensive. A mid-priced material replacing the canvas is a vinyl-coated canvas. The vinyl coated canvas surface cleans easily, costs less than the leather and has great durability. Hanging bags weigh from fifty to 150 pounds, and though the heavier ones move less, they are also less forgiving and more jarring when hit. Floor bags can weigh up to 400 pounds, with most weighing between 150 and 250 pounds. The additional weight is needed to keep the bag from moving when being punched. They are fairly portable, easily placed in an exercise area, and can be purchased at most sporting stores.

There is, however, nothing like training on a hanging bag, being able to have the movement, and hitting with all your power. The bag that meets your needs will depend on your experience, weight, height, and punching strength. A seventy-pound hanging bag is a good starting size for the average person. Some of the bags are filled with water providing a surface that is softer and reducing the jarring kick back of the punch. Other bags are connected on both ends. These are known as double-end heavy bags and are great for beginners.

Hitting the Heavy Bag

It's not just a heavy bag! Imagine you're stepping into the ring with a great champion. Visualize Julio Cesar Chavez rushing out of his corner to defend his title, and give him the fight of his life. If you're a female boxer, see Layla Ali taunting you as she fires jabs and moves away. Cut off the ring and throw combinations. Put passion into your punches and use your imagination, making up combinations, slipping, and circling the bag.

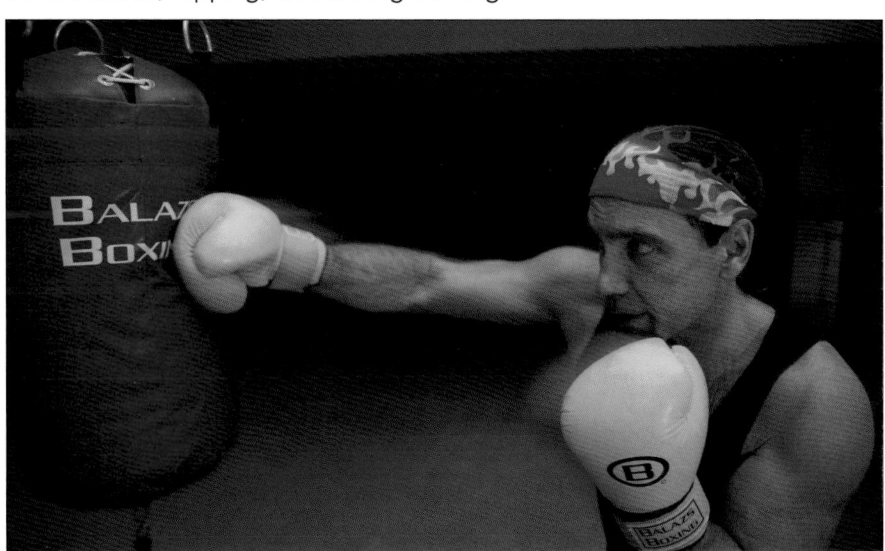

Hitting the heavy bag.

The best part of working out on the heavy bag is that it can be a different workout each and every time, with an endless number of punch combinations being executed. It is an exceptional workout, which can place extreme demands on the musculature, cardiovascular, and respiratory systems. It is creative, fun, and a great way to release tension and stress, giving you a feeling of accomplishment and competence.

The first thing you must do is wrap your hands and put on the gloves. The gloves should feel comfortable, and your hands should fit deeply into them. When the glove makes contact with the bag, the fist should be tight, the wrist straight, and the front of the glove touching the bag. Find your range (the punching distance that you should be away from the bag) for a straight punch by positioning yourself with a fully extended arm at the moment of contact. Hooks and uppercuts require that you stand closer to the bag in order to make contact.

Practice each of the punches until they are mechanically correct, and then add more speed and power. If you are a beginner, work on a single technique for each round, and then mix it up once the movements become second nature. Work the bag as if you were in the ring, moving around and incorporating the back and forth movement of the bag into your workout. When the bag is moving away, step in closer and execute a punch, then back away. Stay light on the feet, including side-to-side movement of the feet and body. Slipping and ducking will help to develop torso strength and teach you about centering the body weight. Pivot the feet when you hit the bag to maintain the balance of the body and to provide a stance from which a maximum power punch can be executed. Never stand flat-footed, but stay on the balls of the feet, ready for movement. To add some power to the jab, step into the punch as it is being delivered.

Develop an action plan for working the bag and have a mental image of your combinations. Experience the workout. It is not a competition to see who can throw the most punches, but a finely orchestrated plan of what punches to throw and how and when to throw those punches.

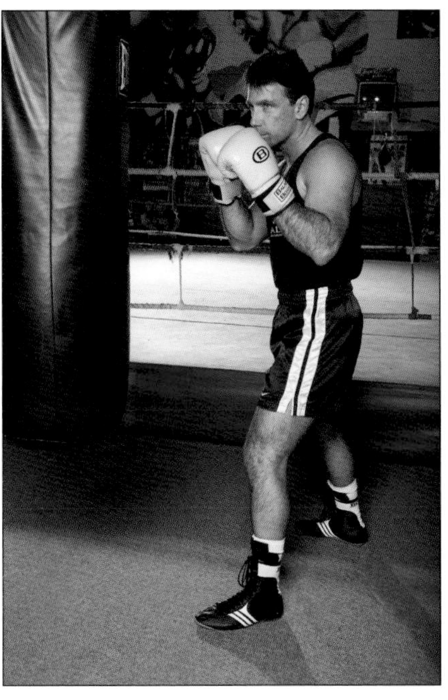

Boxing stance in front of the bag.

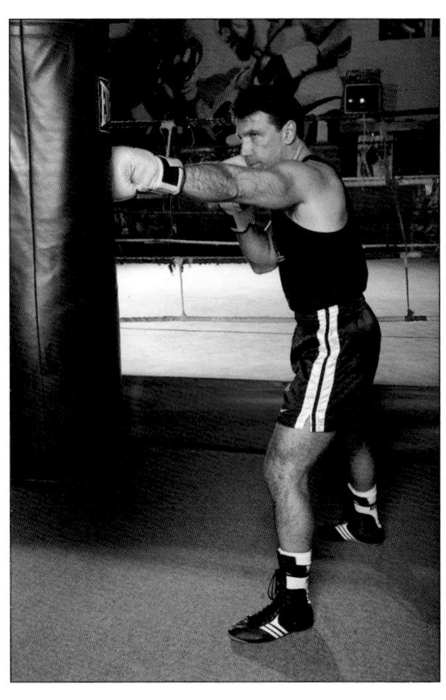

Left jab. Establish your punching range.

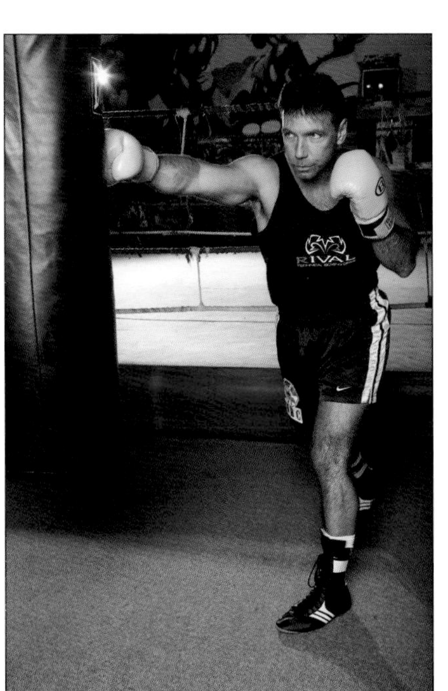

Straight right on the bag.

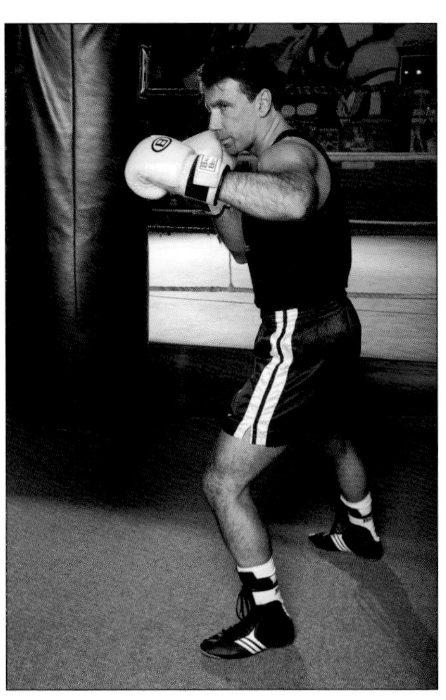

Left hook on the bag.

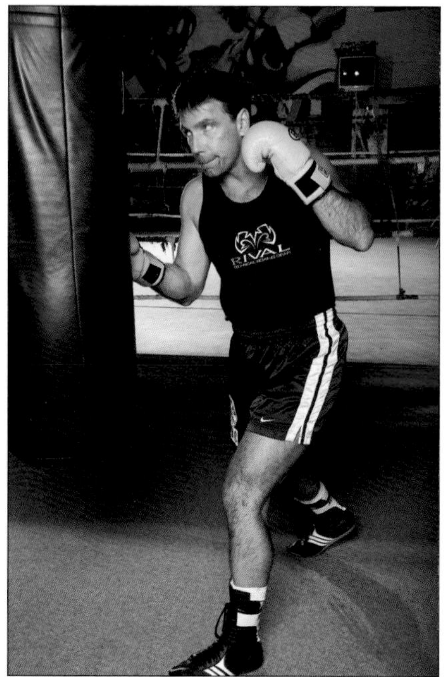

Right uppercut on the bag.

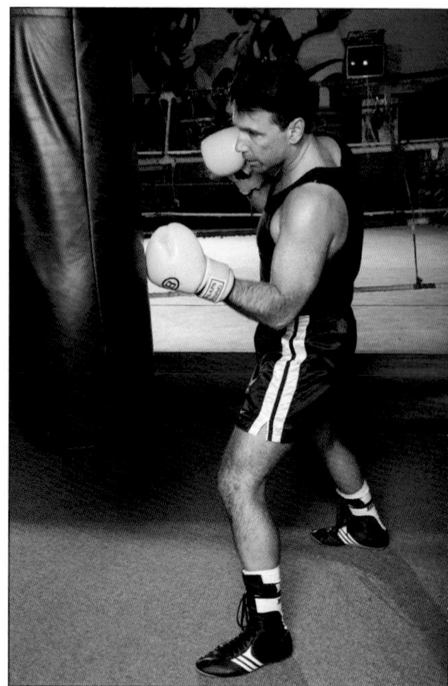

Left uppercut on the bag.

The following steps will assist you in starting to train on the bag. Once you master the basics, move around the bag, attack and retreat, and develop and perfect your own combinations. Remember, use the swinging motion of the bag to your advantage. If the bag is moving away from you, use you legs to get into position to reach the bag. If the bag is swinging towards you, back up and maintain the same punching distance from the bag.

Step 1: Take your boxing stance in front of the bag, always returning to it throughout your workout.

Step 2: Determine your reach or your punching distance. Execute a jab. As you extend the arm, the glove should be in tight contact with the bag. Repeat a few times to get comfortable.

Step 3: Focus and hit in the center of the bag. Mix up the straight punches, a few jabs, and then a straight right.

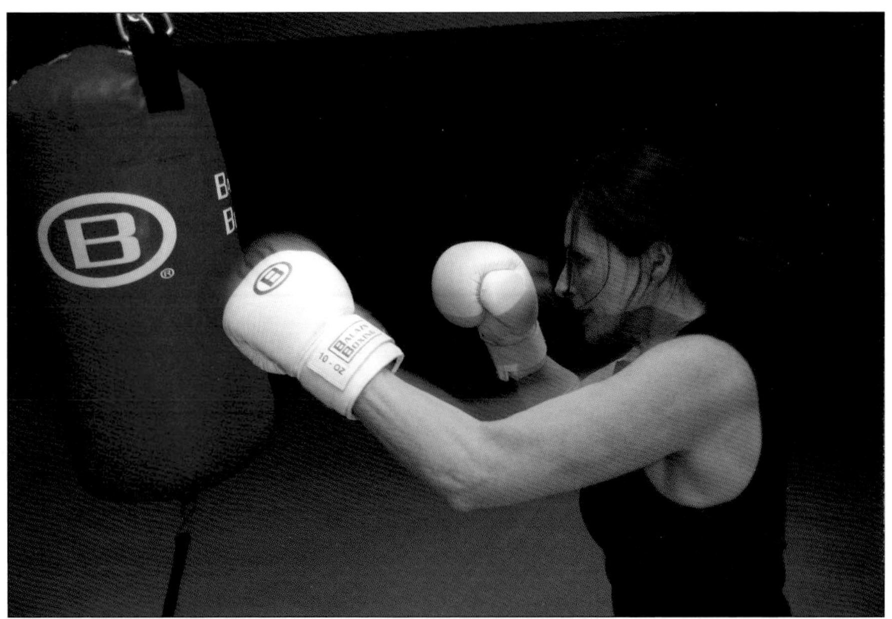

Develop an action plan.

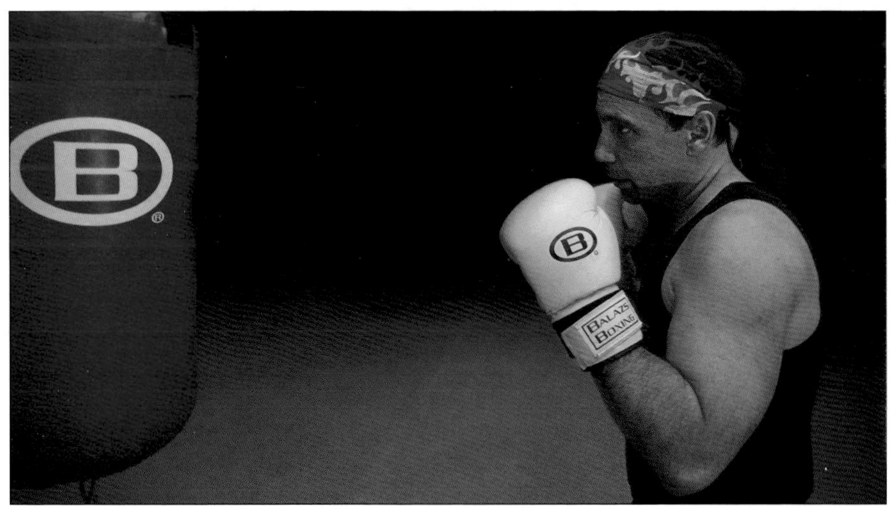

Find your range.

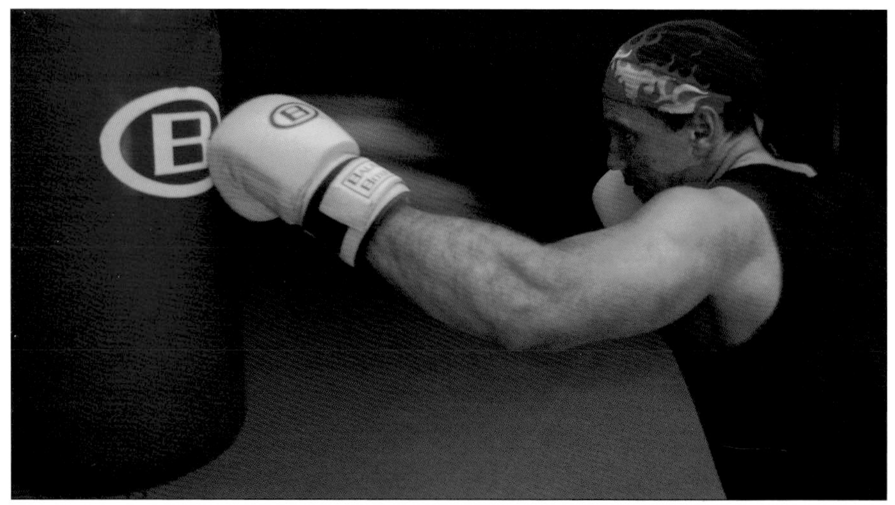

Snap your punches

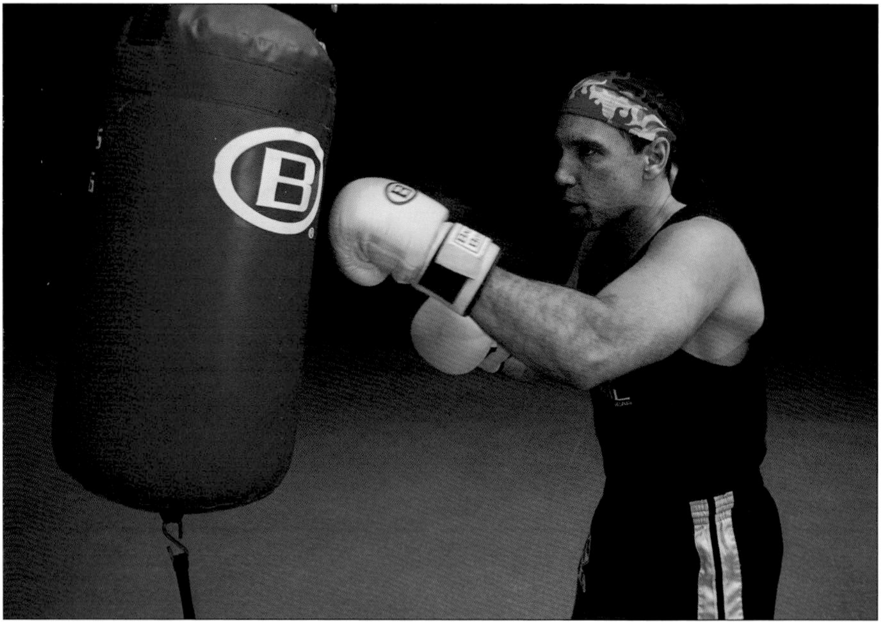

Move around the bag!

Step 4: Next, add movement and more power. Step into the punches and step out. Move the punching hand forward as the front foot moves forward. The hand returns back to the on-guard position as the back foot returns to its original spot.

Step 5: Now, have a plan and mix it up a bit. Move around, slip, and throw a few jabs to determine your reach and target area. Move in closer to the bag, and throw hooks and uppercuts

Beginner Combinations

Double Jabs

Two quick, rapid-fire jabs. It's all about speed. The combination is executed rapidly with a flicking motion on the second jab. The first jab sets the location and has more power behind it. The second is executed by pulling back from the first about one-third of the distance and quickly jabbing. The second punch is meant to catch your opponent off guard.

The One-Two

Throw a left jab followed by a straight right in rapid succession. Slip and move and repeat. (Note: Almost every punch combination should start with the left jab.)

Jab to the Body–Jab to the Head

Step towards the bag and launch a quick left jab to the body, and immediately follow with a jab the head. Move around and circle the bag. Use your legs to lower and raise the height of the jab. You can add a straight right onto this combination: Jab to the body; Jab to the head; throw a quick, straight right; move away; and repeat.

One–Two–Hook

Step into the bag as you launch your left jab, followed by a straight right. You are now in position to throw a short hook to finish the combination. Step away and circle the bag as you plan your next sequence of punches.

Intermediate/Advanced Combinations

One–Two–Hook–Hook

Throw a quick one–two to the body, followed by a left hook to the body, and a left hook to the head (a double left hook). Use your legs to raise or lower the punch height.

Left Jab–Right to the Body–Left Hook to the Jaw

Start with a left jab to the head, lower your body and throw a right under the opponent's guard, moving in at the same time to follow with the left hook. (After the right to the body, the opponent often drops his or her hands, thereby leaving an opening for the third punch, the left hook to the chin.)

Six-Punch Combination

Throw two left jabs (double jab), a straight right, a left hook to the body, a straight right, and then finish with a left jab as you back away from the bag. Try this one slowly, and then speed it up. Move around and repeat.

Flurries

Throw six, seven, or eight rapid-fire punches. Focus on speed rather than power.

Shoe Shining

A succession of quick punches starting at the bottom of the heavy bag working your way up to eye level. This should be at least ten quick punches. Throw this combination in two or three times per round for a challenge.

It is important to start hitting the bag with a plan. If you do not, you will exhaust yourself, risk the chance of injury, and have the feeling of defeat. As with any new activity, learn the technique and build up your stamina to be able to continue the activity. Remember that you are working towards three-minute rounds, so learn to pace your workouts and mix up punches and foot movement.

Heavy Bag Drills

Speed Sprints

An advanced punching workout on the heavy bag involves sprints, which are a succession of fast punches over specified periods of time. The purpose is to increase punch speed, work the arm and back muscles for power and endurance, and challenge the cardiovascular system. This workout imitates the stress placed on the body nearing the end of each round and prepares the muscles to adapt and recover for the next one.

Address the bag straight on, not in a boxing stance, so the arms have equal reach. Maintain this reach distance. Keep the feet stationary, and hold the body core tight. Shift your body weight slightly forward, on the balls of the feet, with knees relaxed. This will give you power and help you focus on throwing punches with speed. Hit the bag in a quick "one-two-one-two" rhythm, fully extending your arms. The sprint times are short, so put a lot of effort into your punches. Breathe naturally throughout the sprints, and punch as fast as possible.

Start with fifteen-second sprints, working up to twenty-five-second sprints. It is best to have a timer. Rest time is equal to sprint time. Walk around and think about your next sprint. Repeat three to four more times.

Burnout Drill

This is a variation on speed sprints. Address the bag straight on. Punch for speed at eye level, alternating the straight left and right punches. Sprint for five seconds, followed by a fifteen-second rest. Ensure you move around the bag, keeping your hands up during the rest period, and sprint again for five seconds. Repeat the five-second sprint, fifteen-second rest for the total three minute round.

Power Drill

This time, you are punching for power instead of speed. In your boxing stance, throw one-twos as hard as you can, starting with five seconds, followed by

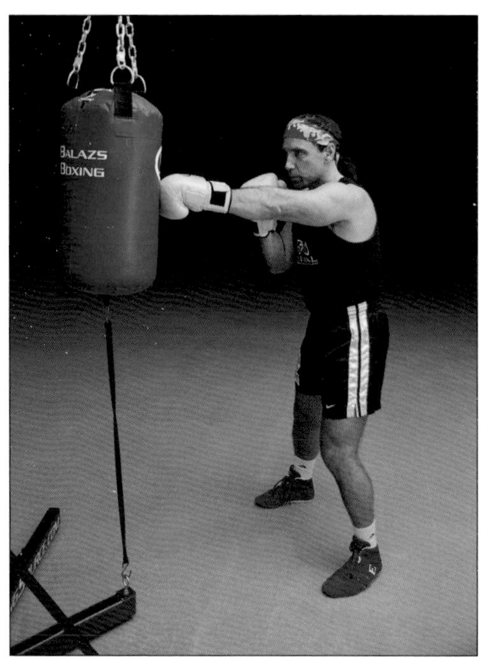

Find your sprinting distance.

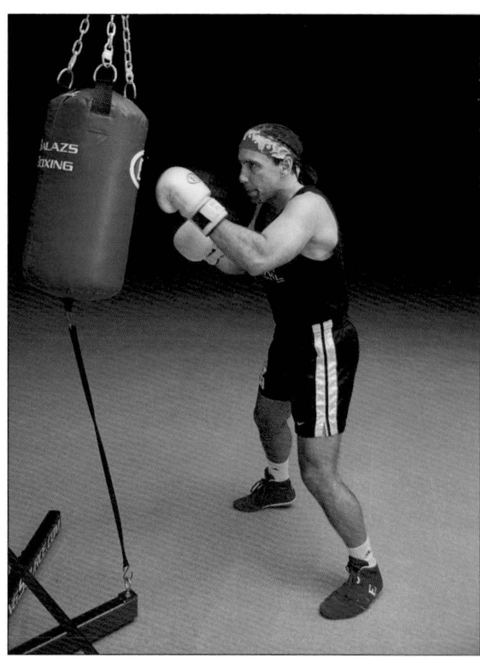

Deliver straight punches, no hooks.

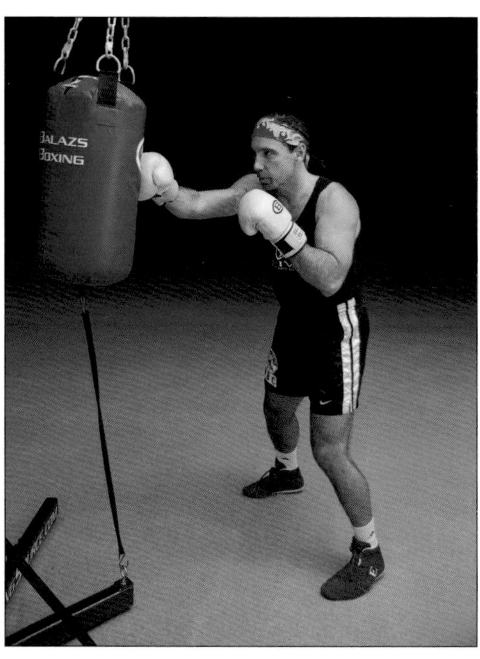

Throw punches as quickly as possible.

a fifteen-second rest, for a total of ninety seconds. Move around the bag, keeping your hands up during the rest period. Try to work your way up to a full three-minute round of power drills, alternating the rest and work intervals.

Speed/Power Sprint

This burnout drill is performed for the last thirty seconds. For the first two and a half minutes, work the bag with punch combinations. For the last thirty seconds, address the bag straight on. Sprint for speed for five seconds as fast as possible and then switch to power sprints for five seconds. Alternate speed sprints and power sprints until the end of the round.

Ladder Drills

Ladder drills are a great way to finish off your heavy bag workout. In the classic boxing stance, throw the left jab, punching at eye level twelve times as fast as possible. Move around and practice slipping and sliding for five to six seconds. Next, jab the bag eleven times, then slip and move around, and so on. Continue all the way down to one repetition. That's ladder one. For ladder two, throw straight rights (throw twelve rights, move around, eleven rights, and move around, and so on.) The third ladder, one-twos (straight left and rights) is even more challenging. Start with twelve one-twos as fast as you can, move around for a few seconds, and repeat all the way down to one repetition.

Common Mistakes and Training Tips:

Mistake: Standing too close to the bag to properly execute a straight punch at maximum power.
Tip: Check your distance before you throw a punch by standing more than a jab length away. Move forward slightly when you throw a jab. Then move back.

Mistake: Pushing the punches on the bag causing the bag to swing excessively. This is often apparent when you get tired.

Tip: As soon as the glove makes contact with the bag, return the arm back to the on-guard position. Snap the punches.

Mistake: The bag spins after it has been hit, revealing an ineffective execution of a punch.
Tip: Strike the bag in the center with the glove and not off to one side.

Mistake: Standing in one place after punching. It is important to include footwork, mix up the punches, and keep the heart rate elevated.
Tip: Move around and circle the bag in between throwing your punches. Move to the right, throw some punches, slip, and move to the left.

Mistake: As fatigue sets in, arms may drop down beside the body, leaving the head unprotected by the fists, which reduces the effectiveness of the punches being thrown.
Tip: Always keep the fists up by the chin protecting the head and the chin.

The Speed Bag

A speed bag is a small punching bag suspended below a platform (horizontal backboard) on a swivel hook, allowing for free rotational movement. It can be mounted on the wall or on a stand. The bags come in various sizes, with the exterior made of stitched leather and the inside filled with a rubber air bladder. The largest speed bags are around fourteen inches long and will move more slowly than the smaller-sized speed bags. The smaller bags (around eight inches) move faster and rebound quickly, making them the most difficult to hit. Working the speed bag develops eye-hand coordination, improves reaction time, rhythm, and upper body endurance. It can be very frustrating initially, but ultimately is fun and worthwhile.

Hitting the Speed Bag

When watching a boxer hit a speed bag, one wonders, "How can you make contact with something moving that fast?" And if you listen, it is the sound of the rhythm of the bag hitting the backboard that inspires one hand moving

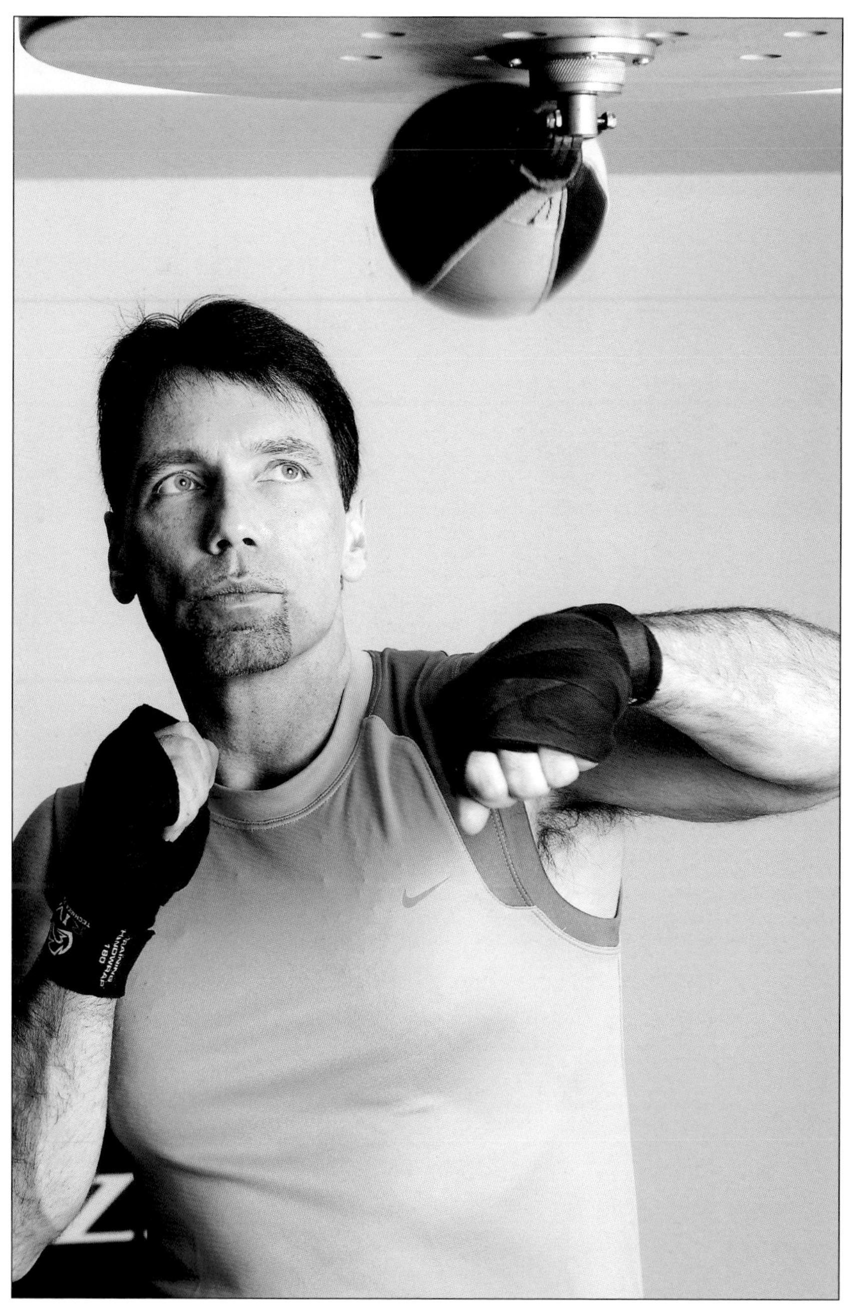

Hitting the speed bag.

over the other to make contact with the bag. There are actually three sounds on the backboard that you hear. Stand facing the bag, strike the bag, and it will move directly away from you and make contact with the back of the platform (sound #1). The bag will rebound towards you and hit the front of the platform (sound #2). The bag then returns to hit the back of the platform (sound #3) and you must get ready: As the bag rebounds forward, it is your turn to strike it once again. The rhythm is "punch –1-2–3". You hit the bag; the bag hits the platform back, front, and back.

The surface of your knuckles making contact with the bag and how hard you hit it will influence your ability to keep the bag under control and in the "punch-1-2-3" rhythm. Start with one hand, using medium force until you have mastered the rhythm; then add the speed and power, alternating the hands. Hand wraps give the basic protection required. Or if your hands are sensitive, use speed-bag striking mitts.

Step 1: Face the speed bag, so it is square with the body. Bring both fists up and in front of the face. This is the one time you do not have to be in the boxer's stance. The bottom of the bag should be one to two inches above chin level for the larger bags and eye level for the smaller bags. Adjust the speed-bag height to the appropriate level. If it is non-movable, find a step to stand on.

Step 2: Strike the bag in the center near the bottom edge, making sure the knuckles land flush against the leather. Hit straight on and straight through the bag. Don't chop at the bag. Visualize hitting through the bag, and then bring the fist back to the starting position.

Step 3: Repeat striking the bag with the "punch-1-2-3" rhythm, keeping both hands up by the face. Work with one fist, then the other, taking the arm through a circular motion. As you punch faster, tighten up this circular range of motion that the arm goes through.

Step 4: Go slowly at first, and if the bag is moving too fast, let some air out of the bladder to slow it down or try a larger bag. The bag will appear to have a

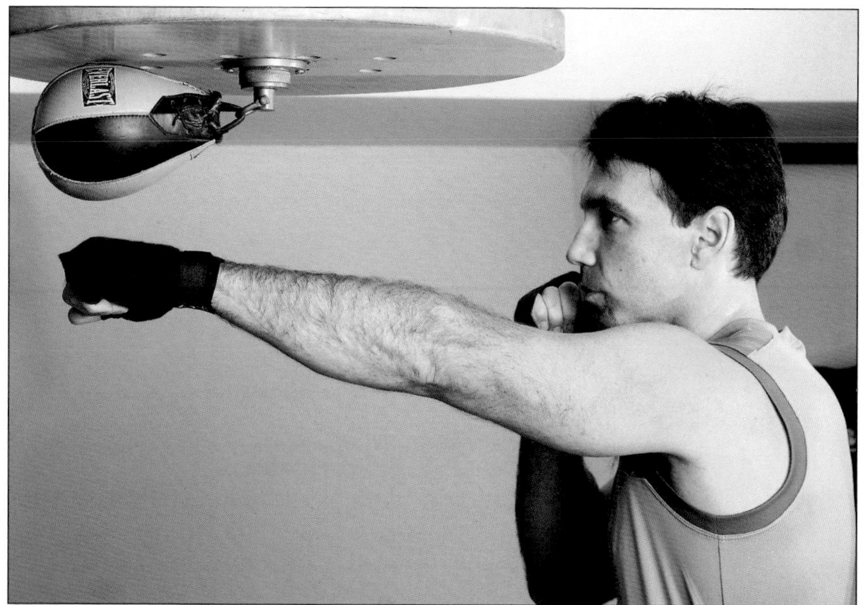

Make contact with the knuckles.

mind of its own and may either moves in circles or not respond to your strike. It's all a matter of timing. If you make contact too soon, you will jam the movement of the bag. If contact is made too late, your fist will strike the underside of the bag and cause a clumsy rhythm.

Step 5: Strike the speed bag four times with your right fist and then four times with your left fist, eventually taking it to two strikes with each fist. Once you have mastered the doubles, try making single strikes. This is called a two-handed rhythm and requires that one fist is brought up behind and over the top of the other. For example, as you strike the speed bag with your left fist, bring the right fist up behind and over the top of the left fist, and then strike the bag with the right fist. Repeat, keeping the semi-circular movement short and fast.

Step 6: Nothing in boxing remains stationary. To remind yourself of this, and to increase the challenge, move around the bag as you practice your combinations. Remember, always train the way you intend to perform.

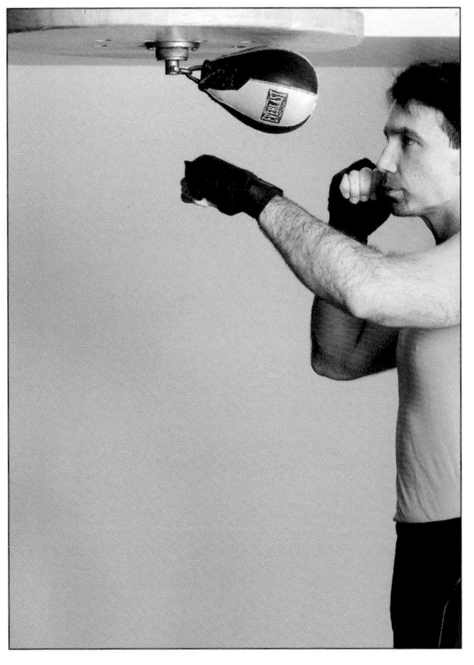

Bag rebounds to hit front platform.

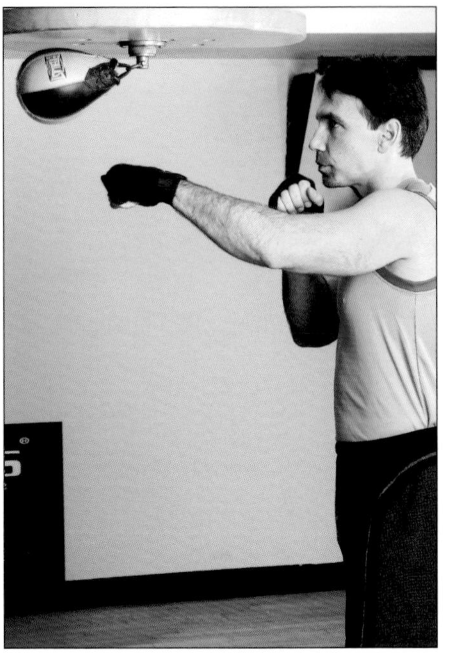

Follow through with your punch.

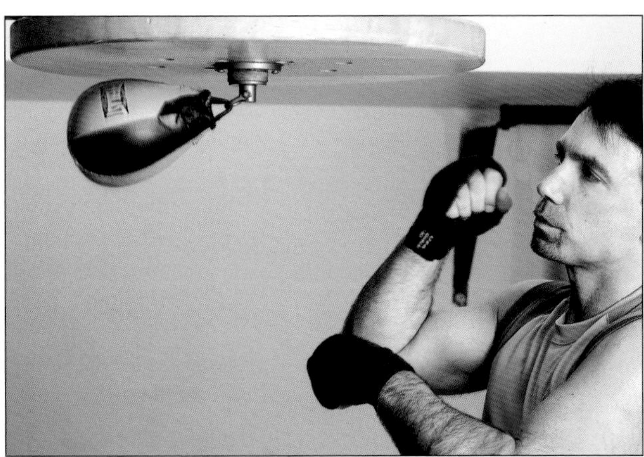

Repeat striking in a 1-2-3 rhythm.

Speed Bag Combinations:

- Single punches: Punch, alternating hands.
- Double punches: Double punches, alternating hands.
- Double Punches with movement–Alternate double punches with each hand: while stepping around to the left and to the right side.

Common Mistakes & Teaching Tips:

Mistake: Striking the bag too hard, making the bag spin and move erratically.
Tip: Slow down the punch movement. Hit it lightly at first. Make sure the circular movement is not too large and that the fists do not drop down below chest level in order to maintain a steady rhythm.

Mistake: Striking the speed bag with the side of the fist.
Tip: Striking with the side of the fist is a more advanced move. For beginners, the knuckle portion of the fist should make contact with the bag. Rotate the fist just before contacting the bag.

Mistake: Standing slightly sideways or in the boxing stance when hitting the bag.
Tip: Always stand square to the bag to ensure that both arms have equal reach.

Work up to hitting the bag with single strikes and increase speed. Use a smaller speed bag to challenge and improve your agility and eye-hand coordination. Vary the speed of the punches (slower punches interspersed with sprints. Once you have your rhythm down, move around the bag while punching).

The Double-End Striking Bag

No need for a sparring partner when you have a double-end striking bag.

The double-end striking bag comes in a number of sizes, much like the speed bag, and has an air-filled bladder. Generally made out of leather, it can also be constructed with vinyl-coated canvas. A rope suspends the bag on

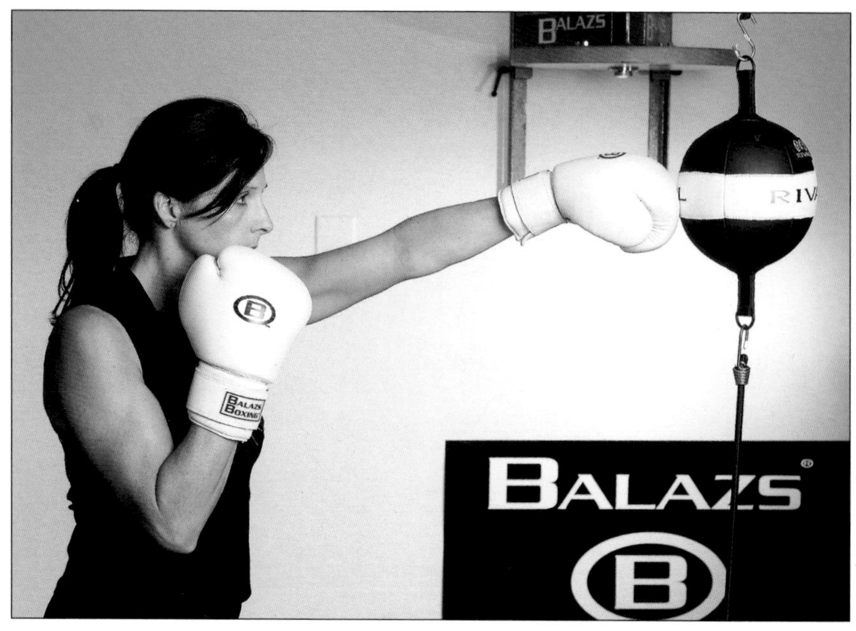

Strike the bag in the center.

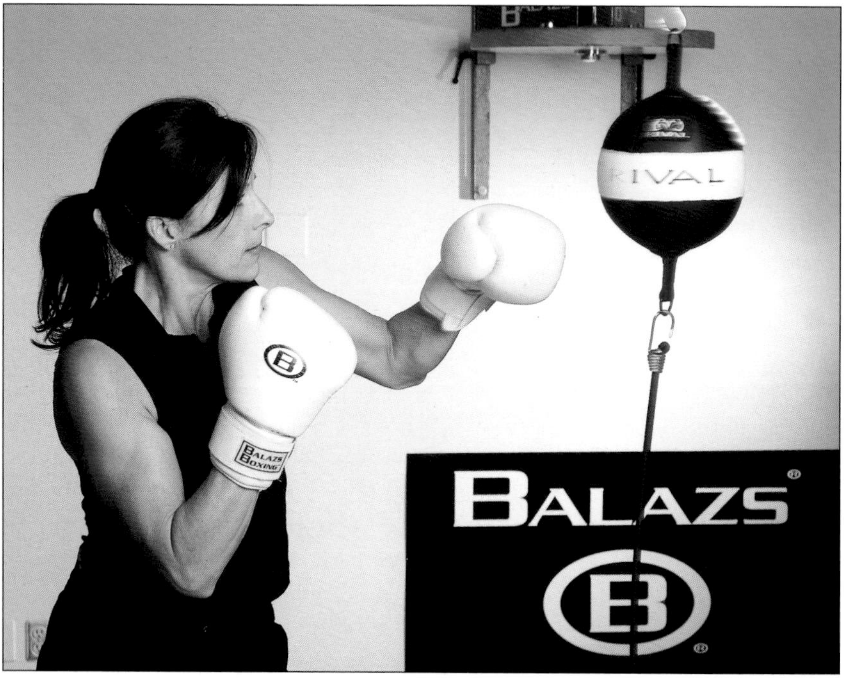

Strike the bag with the left jab.

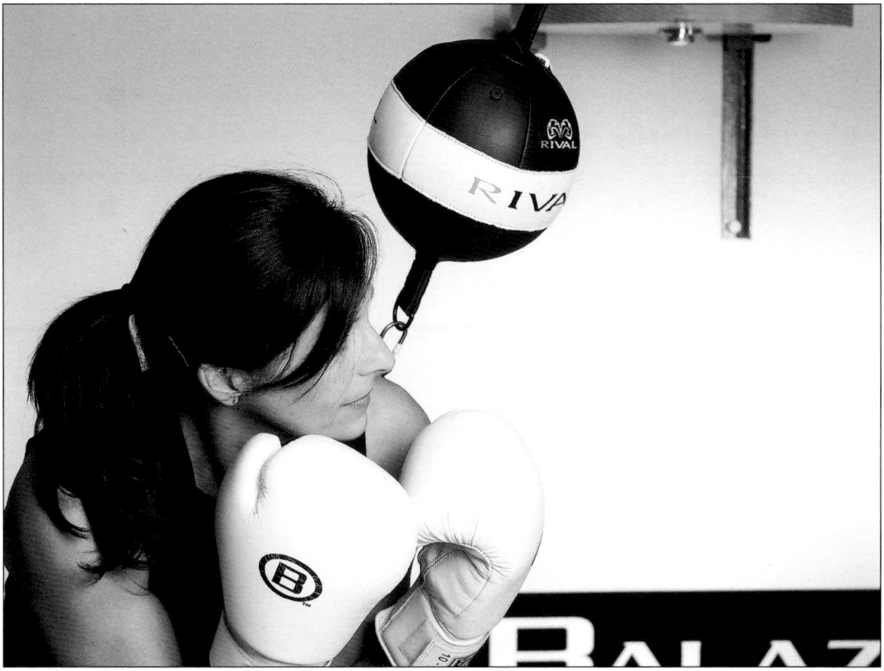

Slip the rebound to the right.

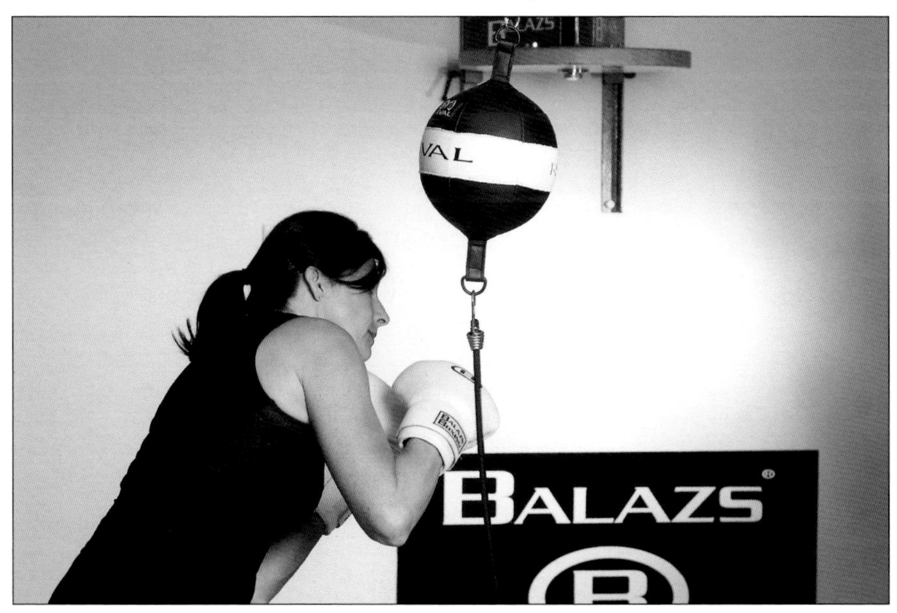

Slip the rebound to the left.

the top and an elastic shock cord holds the bottom to give an unforgiving rebound action when it is hit. Because the surface is so much smaller than that of the heavy bag, the double-end striking bag challenges your eye-hand coordination. Instead of focusing on power, these punches are intended to improve coordination, reactions, timing, and agility. You can either wear your bag gloves or hand wraps when hitting the double-end striking bag. Because boxing gloves give a larger contact surface, slowing the bag movement, they initially may be a better choice when starting.

There is an entirely different rhythm to hitting the double-end bag than any other bags. Heavy bags don't punch back; double-end bags do! You learn to bob and weave, slip and duck, keep your hands up, and move your head. When you strike the double-end bag, it will move quickly away and then rebound back at you.

Step 1: Address the bag in your boxing stance. Keep your hands up, and get ready to move. Stay light on your feet, the weight centered towards the balls of the feet.

Step 2: Strike the bag with a left jab, and as the bag rebounds, slip to the right, quickly returning to your upright stance, (classic boxing stance). Continue practicing this one punch until you have mastered the movement. Work on technique, not power. Strike the center of the bag, making the bag move directly back and straight at you. Move out of the way, and then strike the bag again.

Combinations:

Left Jab

(Jab-slip right.) Snap a left jab. As the bag starts to rebound, quickly slip to the right, and then move back into position, ready to throw your next punch. Repeat practicing the jab and slip until you find your rhythm.

Double Jabs

(Double Jab-slip right.) Throw two quick jabs and then slip to the right as the bag fully rebounds.

One-Two Combo

(One-two-slip left.) Throw a quick one-two together (no full rebound of the bag between the left jab and straight right) and then slip to the left side.

Advanced Combo

(Jab-jab-straight right-slip right-slip-left-one-two.) Throw a double jab, straight right, slip right, slip left as the bag fully rebounds and finish with a one-two punch.

Common Mistakes and Teaching Tips:

Mistake: Hitting the side of the bag, causing it to rotate.
Tip: Focus on striking the bag flush in the center.

Mistake: Hitting the bag with too much power, causing the bag to rebound ineffectively.
Tip: Focusing on throwing quick, light punches. Save the power and the strength for the heavy bag.

Mistake: The slips are exaggerated, moving the body more than needed, causing an off-balance situation.
Tip: Practice moving only the head and shoulders just enough to avoid the rebound of the bag. Focus on balance, leaning to the side, staying on the balls of the feet, never leaning back.

Practice your slips, add footwork, move in and out, circle the bag, and mix up the punches. Be sure to include rapid-succession punching, combinations, and defensive moves. Always remember to keep the fists up by the chin, the elbows close to body, and the eyes on the target. Plan your next move.

Mitt Work

5

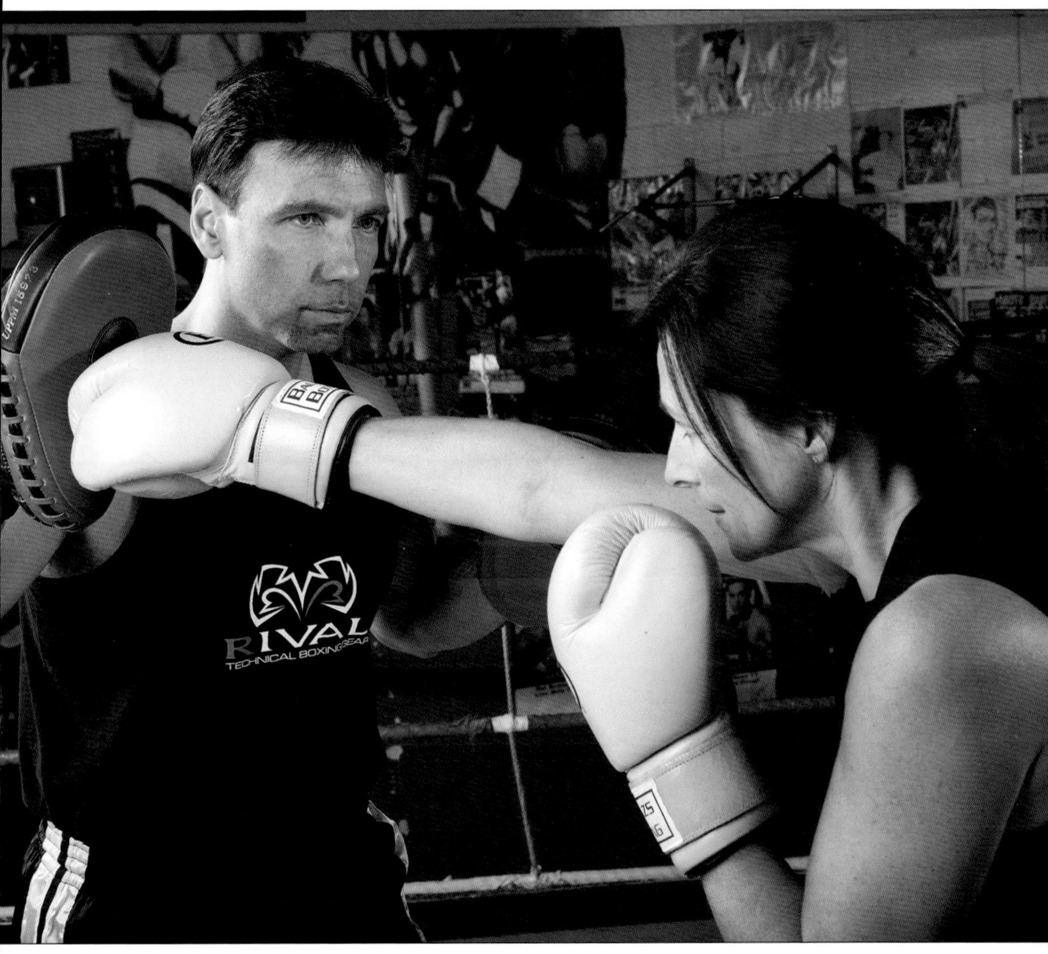

Target Mitts

The Basics

Training with target mitts is the next best thing to actually sparring. It's a great way to improve your punching speed and accuracy. At first, the punches should be light and the technical execution is of prime importance. The puncher will learn to react quickly and effectively. Improving the strength and power of your punches should be developed on the heavy bag.

There are two roles when training with target mitts: The person holding the mitts and calling out the punch commands is called the "catcher" and the person throwing is called the "puncher."

The Catcher

The catcher wears the target mitts and controls the action by calling out punch combinations. The target mitts are held about two feet away from the body, arms slightly bent at the elbow in a semi-tense position. The legs and feet are in a classic boxing stance to add stability to receive the punches and the body core (torso) is kept tight and strong. The puncher must always be kept in view. When catching, keep the elbows bent slightly because this helps to absorb the impact of the punch.

The Puncher

The puncher stands in front of the catcher, in the classic boxing stance ready to execute a punch, and stays slightly more than a jab-length away, always watching the target and listening for the catcher's commands.

Throw punches with the purpose of improving technique, accuracy, and speed. The idea is to get the feel of throwing an accurate and efficient punch.

When starting, the catcher calls for the basic straight punches. Assuming the puncher is in the classic boxing stance, all jabs (left hand) are thrown at the catcher's left-hand target mitt. All straight rights are thrown at the catcher's right-hand target mitt. Left hooks should be thrown at the catchers left target mitt. The catcher must turn the mitt inward to receive this punch. Right uppercuts are thrown to the right target mitt, and left uppercuts are thrown to the left target mitt. The catcher must turn the target mitt down to be able to catch this punch. Having the puncher throw across to the opposite target mitt helps to keep the punches straight in front of the body. It also helps to develop a slight rotation in the upper body to assist the execution of the punches and in strengthening of the torso.

Add combinations once the puncher is comfortable with accuracy and responding quickly. The catcher should remind the puncher to focus on technique instead of power and to keep at least a jab-length away. Once you both become comfortable with the basic punches, add footwork and movement forward, backward, and side to side. The puncher must wait until he or she receives the punch commands from the catcher to ensure the catcher is in the ready position to receive the punches. Remember, the catcher sets the pace of the round. When catching, be sure to move the mitt forward slightly to meet the incoming punch. This minimizes impact on the shoulder joint.

Beginner Drills

Drill One

Twenty left jabs. (Catcher gets ready to receive jabs and counts the punches. This is not a sprint. The puncher steps in, snaps a jab, and moves around.)

Drill Two

Twenty straight rights. (Catcher gets ready to receive straight rights, and counts. This is not a sprint. The puncher steps in, snaps a straight right, and moves around.)

Drill Three

20 one-twos. Left jab, straight right.

These drills need to be practiced until both the catcher and the puncher feel comfortable and are working together. Focus on one- and two-punch combinations before moving into multiple-punch combinations.

Building Combinations

The catcher calls out the following number(s) to indicate what punch to throw:

1: Left jab

2: Straight right

3: Left hook

4: Right uppercut

Catcher calls 1: Puncher throws a left jab.

Catcher calls 2: Puncher throws a straight right.

Catcher calls 1-2: Puncher throws a left jab-straight right combination.

Catcher calls 1-2-3: Puncher throws a left jab-straight right-left hook combination.

Catcher calls 1-2-3-4: Puncher throws a left jab-straight right-left hook-right uppercut combination.

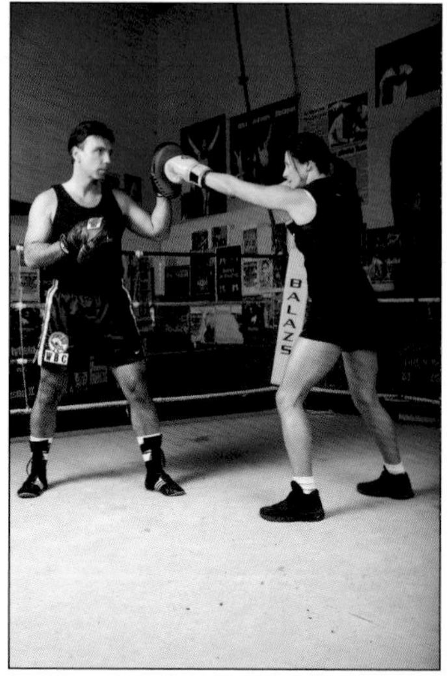

Puncher delivers the left jab to the catcher's left mitt.

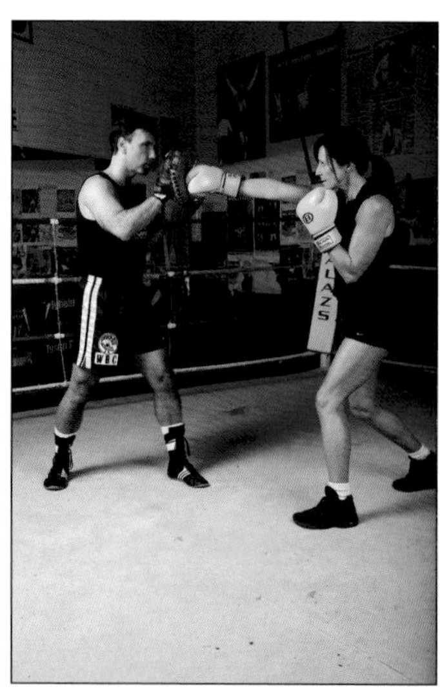

Puncher delivers straight right to catcher's right mitt.

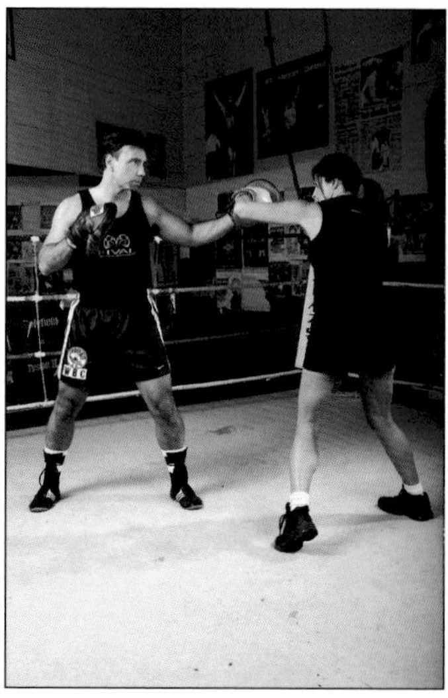

Catcher turns left mitt inward to receive the left hook.

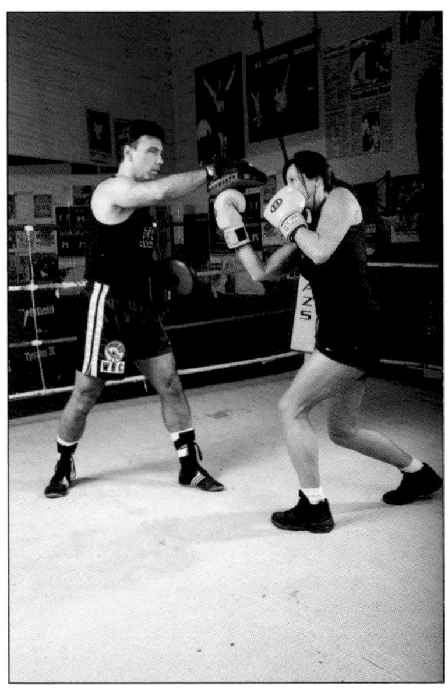

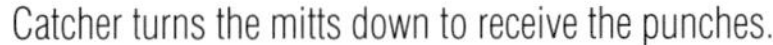

Catcher turns the mitts down to receive the punches.

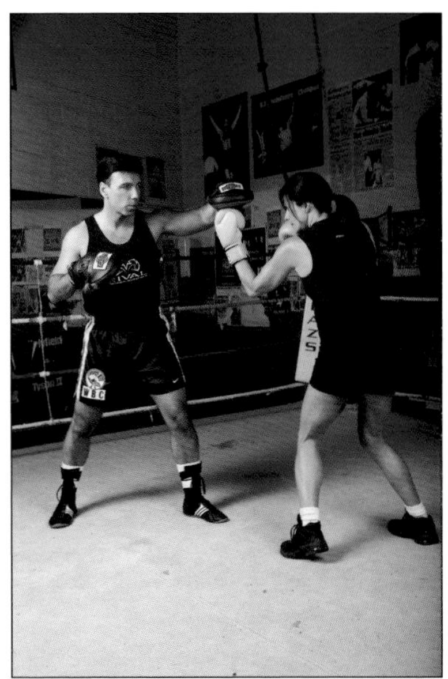

Left uppercut.

It is suggested to train on the basic target mitt drills for a number of workouts. It takes several weeks to build the eye-hand coordination and punching/catching techniques on target mitts to ensure you are ready for the more advanced drills.

Common Mistakes and Tips

Mistake: The puncher is standing too close to the catcher, thereby not being able to execute the punches correctly.
Tip: The catcher should remind the puncher to back up after throwing a punch or series of punches. Punch and get out.

Mistake: The catcher holds the target mitts with straight arms.
Tip: The catcher must keep the arms slightly bent at the elbow joint, allowing the arms to absorb the punch. Remember to move the mitt forward slightly to meet the incoming punch.

Mistake: Throwing punches too hard, leading to improper technique.
Tip: The purpose of target mitt training is to improve technique, speed, accuracy, and reaction time. Greater power comes from better technique. Save the hard punches for the heavy bag.

Mistake: The catcher and the puncher are not working together. The catcher may not be focused on the puncher and the placement of the punches. The puncher throws punches and does not wait for instructions from the catcher.
Tip: The catcher should have a game plan and be aware of what is going on. You set the tempo. Clearly communicate the combination you want executed.

Advanced Target Mitts

Target mitts allow you to work on offensive and defensive moves while practicing specific drills. It's a step up from bag work since the target is capable of moving and reacting. Once you have your range and feel comfortable with the basic combinations, start to incorporate more advanced drills.

Defensive Moves

Including defensive moves to target mitt training adds a sense of realism and makes for a challenging workout. There are three defensive techniques that you need to understand and practice: Blocking, parrying, and slipping a punch. These defensive moves are integral to the advanced target mitt drills.

Blocking

Blocking guards the head and body from the impact of a punch and displaces some of the force of that punch. Straight punches to the head are blocked by holding the fist and the inside portion of the glove high by the face. To block incoming punches to the body, the shoulders, forearms, and elbows are positioned to prevent contact from the incoming punch by being placed between the glove and the body core. When the punch meets your gloves, absorb some of the force of the punch by bending a little at the waist and the knees. The puncher needs to stay relaxed, knowing that there will be contact.

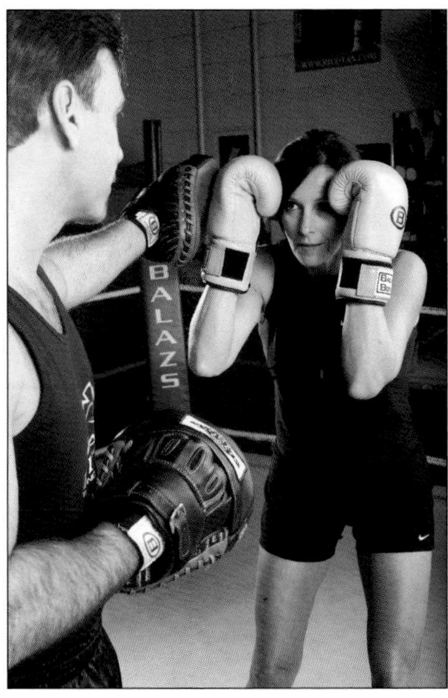

Puncher holds hands high in on-guard position.

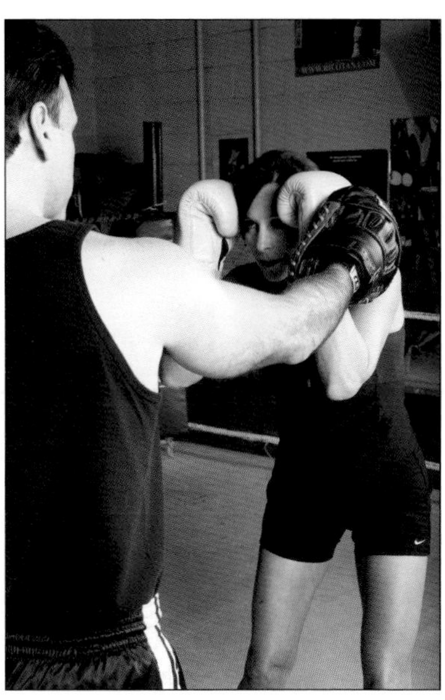

Catcher simulates a left and right hook. Puncher blocks punches.

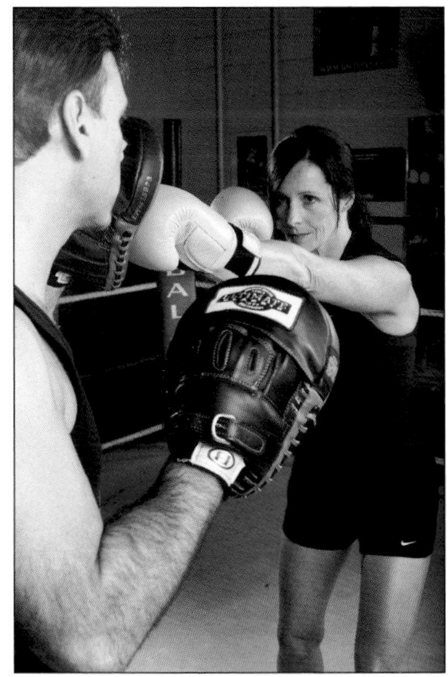

Puncher throws a left jab.

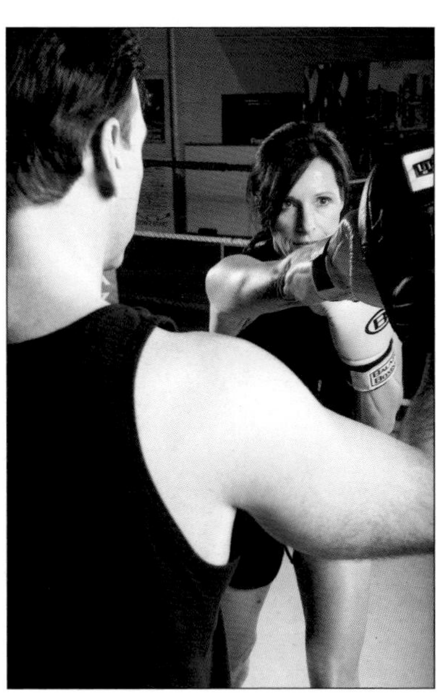

Puncher throws a straight right.

Blocking Combination: Block/Block – 1-2

The puncher holds hands high in on-guard position, keeping the gloves tight against the head. The catcher simulates a left and right hook by lightly tapping the puncher's gloves with the inside (cushion side) of the mitt—left then right mitt. The puncher blocks both punches and then fires back with a quick 1-2 (left-right) to the target mitts.

Common Mistakes and Training Tips

Mistake: The catcher throws too hard.
Tip: The contact from the catcher should be a tap on the glove of the puncher.

Mistake: The puncher pulls hands away from his or her head when blocking.
Tip: The puncher must keep the hands up close and tight to the head when blocking to avoid being hit with his or her own gloves.

Parrying

Parrying or catching a punch means that the punch is deflected or redirected. To parry a punch, "catch" the punch with the palm side of your glove and then deflect it. Keep your gloves up high while you wait for the punch to come in. To parry an incoming left jab, use the inside of your right glove. To parry a straight right, use the inside of your left glove. Parrying is more effective than blocking a straight punch because the punch is redirected and not just neutralized. By redirecting the momentum of the incoming punch, openings may be created for counterpunches. Reaching or pawing at an incoming punch is a common mistake, so wait for the punch before you catch it.

Parrying Combination: Parry/Jab

The catcher simulates a left jab by throwing a punch towards the puncher's gloves (head area). The puncher parries or catches the jab with the inside or palm portion of the right glove, keeping the left hand free for a potential left jab counterpunch. The catcher throws a slow jab at three-quarters speed, so

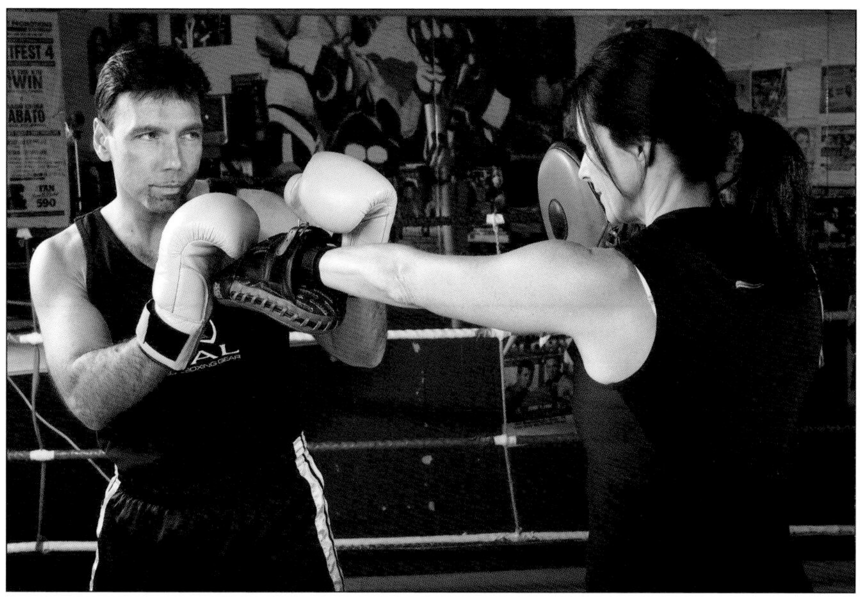

Catcher parries a punch.

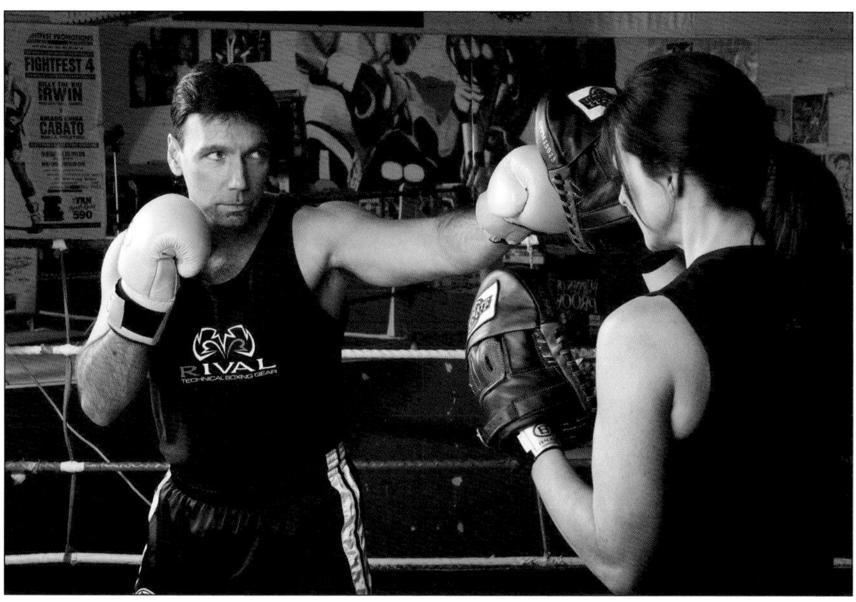

Puncher throws a left jab.

the puncher has time to see it coming. Once both partners are comfortable parrying the jab, the puncher can add a counter jab back to the target mitts. It's very important to communicate and work together. Increase the speed of this when ready.

Common Mistake and Training Tip

Mistake: Pawing, reaching, or slapping at an incoming straight punch, leaving your head exposed.
Tip: Wait and calculate the correct time to deflect and redirect the incoming punch.

Slipping

Slipping is an effective defensive technique, but also the most difficult to learn. You must react sooner to slip the punch because your entire body is moving to avoid the incoming punch.

To slip punches, practice bending slightly at the waist and knees, moving the body to the left or the right, so that the punches miss you. Slip only enough to avoid the punch, staying balanced, ready to counterpunch. Keep your hands up to protect your head, in case the slip was not effective, and be in a set position for the counterpunch. To slip a left jab, lean your body and move your head and shoulders to the right. To slip a straight right, lean your body and move your head and shoulders to the left. Always return to your classic boxing stance as quickly as possible. Slipping punches leaves both hands completely open to counterpunching unlike parrying and blocking.

Slipping Combination: Slip/Slip – 1-2

The catcher throws a left jab aiming for the puncher's left shoulder. The puncher "slips" to the right to avoid the punch. Work on this move until the puncher is comfortable slipping the left jab. Now practice slipping the straight right. The catcher throws a straight right aiming for the puncher's right shoulder. The puncher "slips" to the left to avoid the punch.

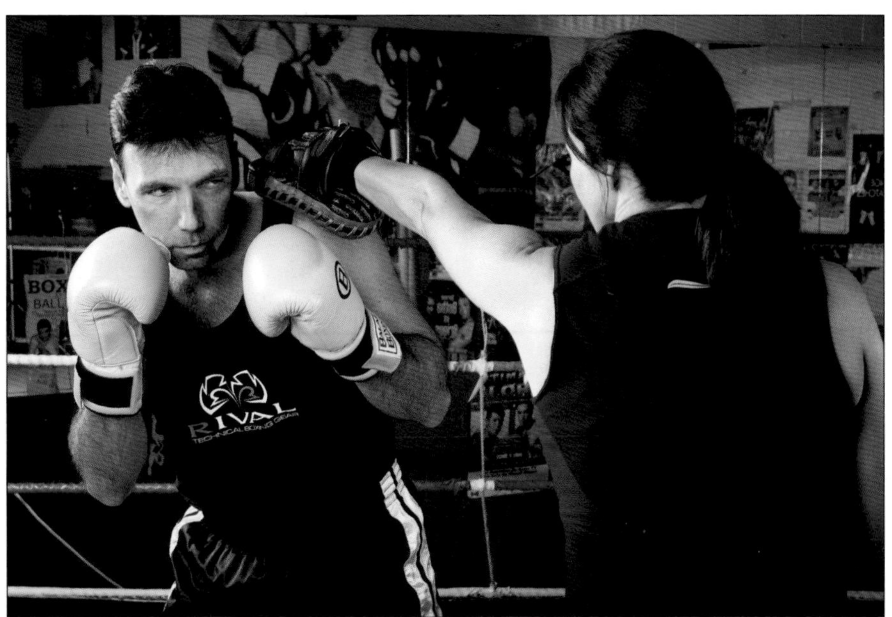

Slip to the right.

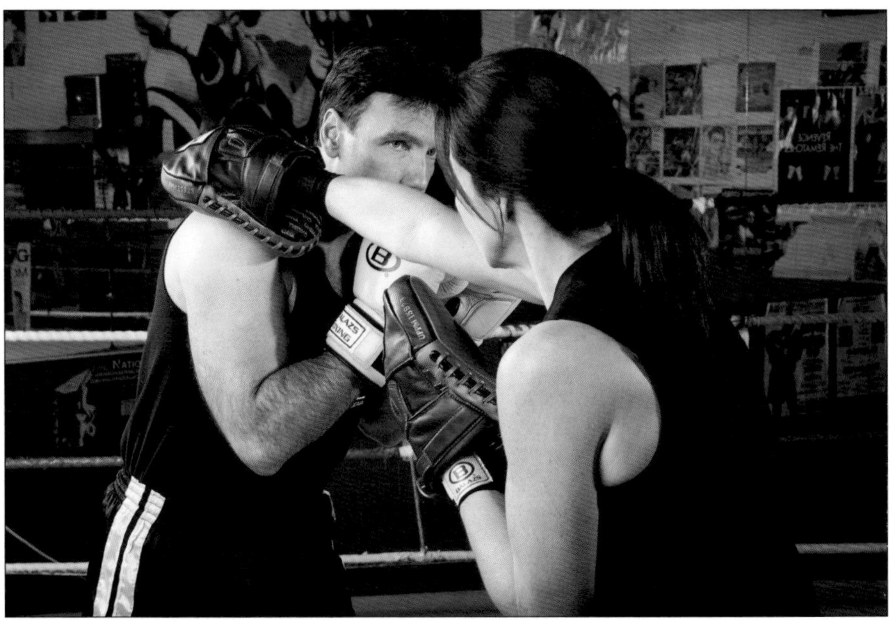

Slip to the left.

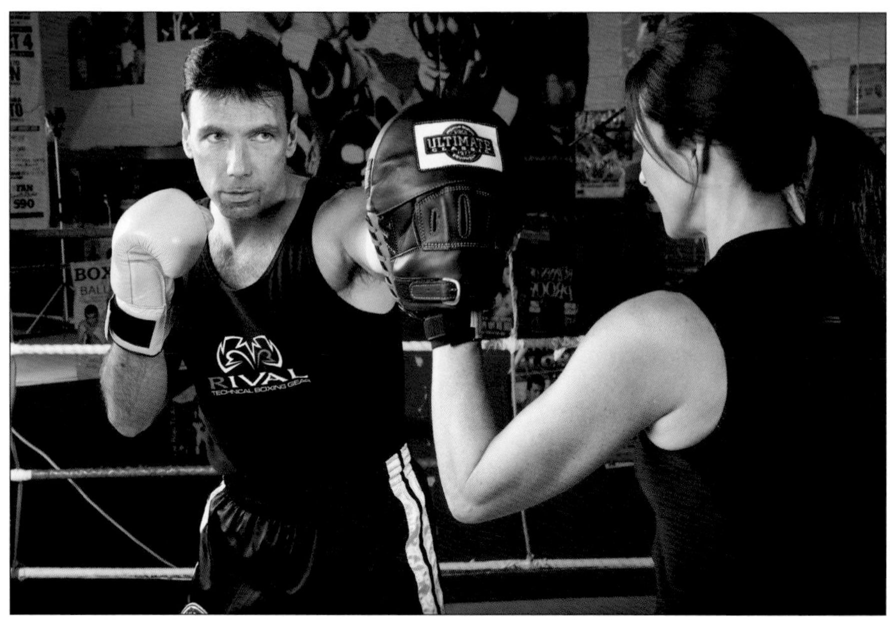

Puncher throws a left jab.

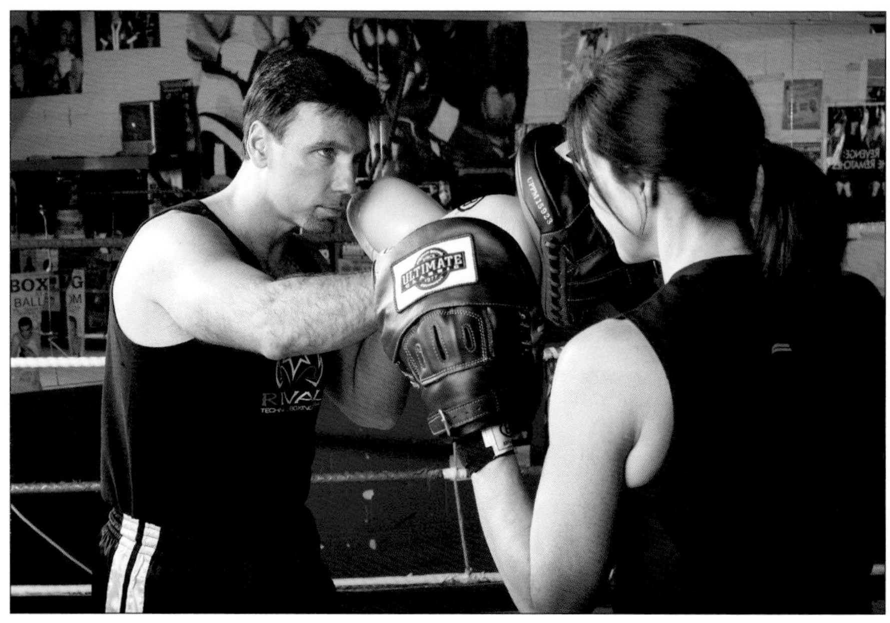

Puncher throws a straight right.

Once you have the hang of this, add some punches to the combination. The catcher throws a 1-2 (left-right). The puncher slips to the right, then left, avoiding both punches. The puncher follows up with a 1-2 (left-right) of his own to the target mitts.

Common Mistakes and Training Tips

Mistake: Overslipping, causing the body to be off balanced and out of position. This may put you on the back of your heels instead of on the balls of your feet.
Tip: Practice in front a mirror. Stay on the balls of the feet and focus on your center of balance.

Mistake: Taking your eyes off of your partner or looking at the floor.
Tip: Always keep your eyes on your partner in order to respond quickly.

Building Advanced Combinations

Combination One: Parry/Jab-Jab – Slip/Right Cross

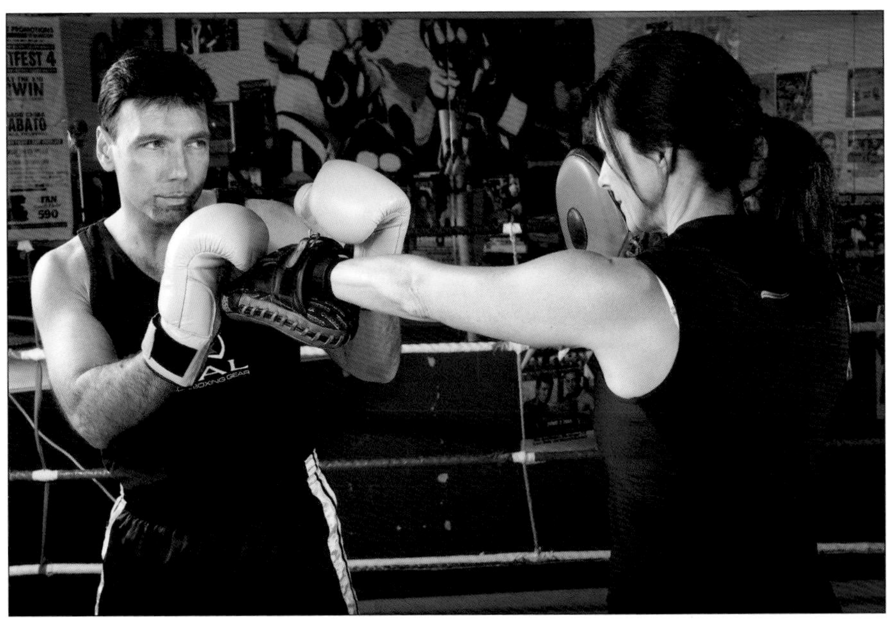

Parry

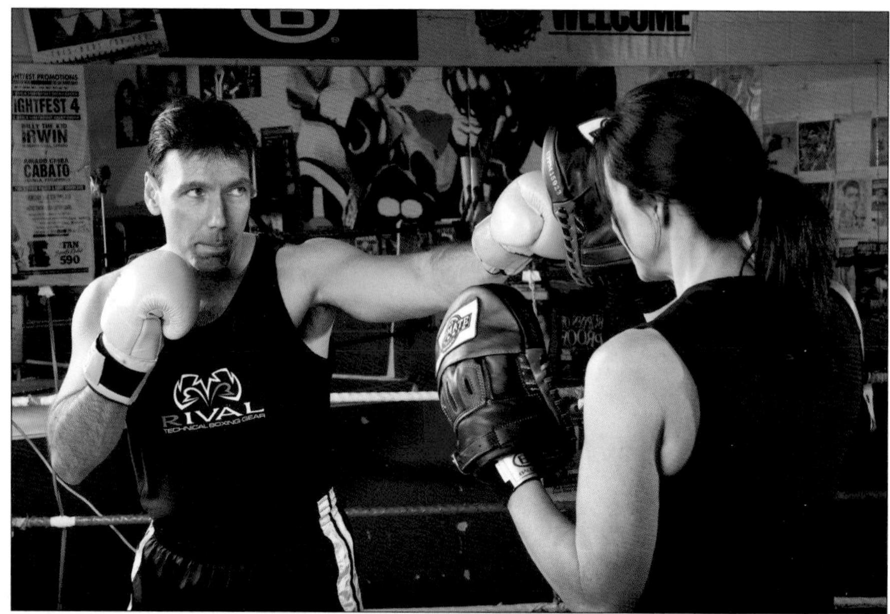
IRWIN
CABATO
590
RIVAL
TECHNICAL BOXING GEAR

Jab

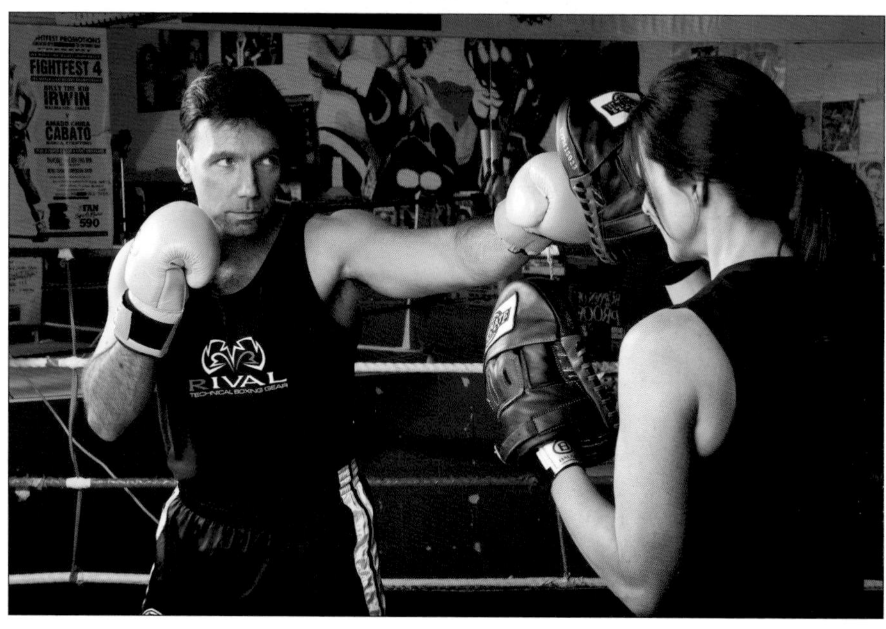
FIGHTFEST 4
IRWIN
CABATO
590
RIVAL
TECHNICAL BOXING GEAR

Jab

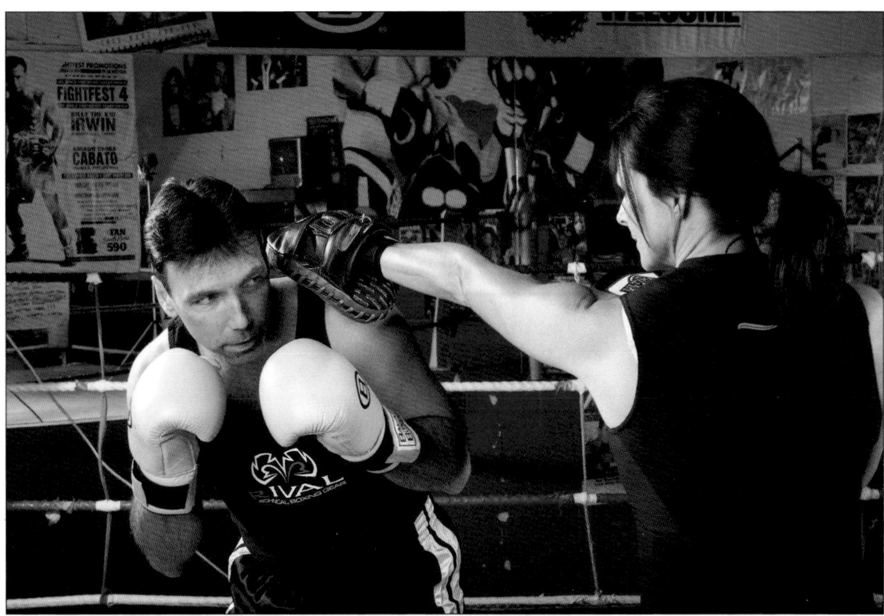

Slip

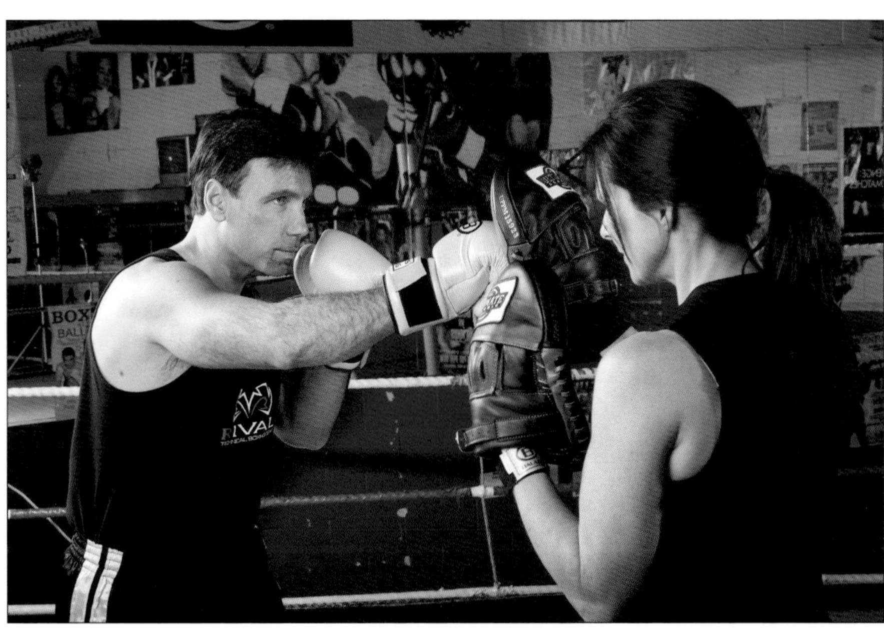

Right Cross

Step 1: The catcher simulates a jab, the puncher parries the jab and throws two quick jabs back (the catcher throws at three-quarters speed). Parry/jab-jab. Repeat several times.
Step 2: Slip/right Cross: Catcher throws a jab, puncher slips to the right side, and counters with a right.
Step 3: Put it all together: Catch a jab with the right hand (parry) and immediately throw two jabs. Slip the second jab and throw a right cross.

Combination Two: Slip/Uppercut–Slip/Hook

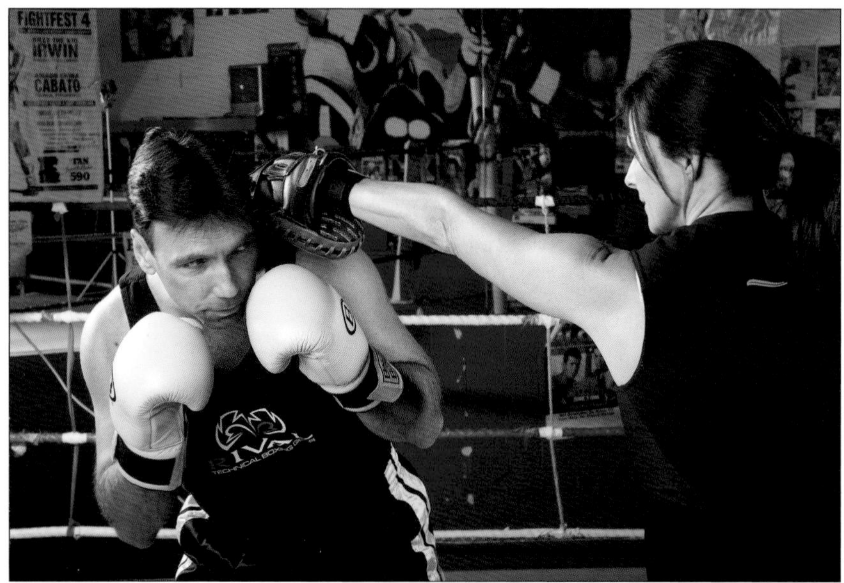

Slip

Step 1: Slip/Uppercut: The catcher throws a left jab, the puncher slips right, (the puncher slips a left jab) and then throws a right uppercut. Practice this five or six times.
Step 2: Slip/hook: The catcher throws a straight right, and the puncher slips to the left and counterpunches with a left hook.
Step 3: Put it all together: Slip/uppercut–slip/hook.

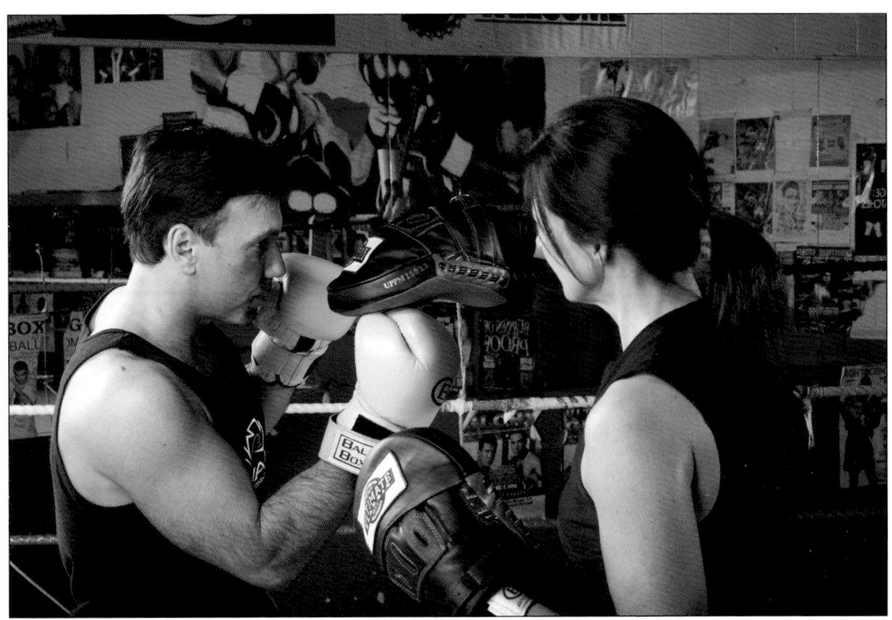

Uppercut

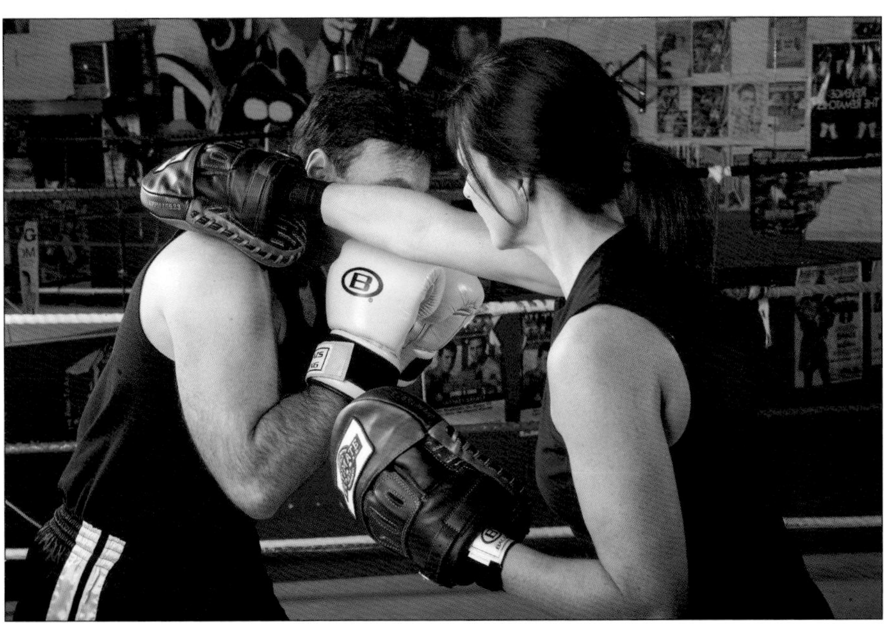

Slip

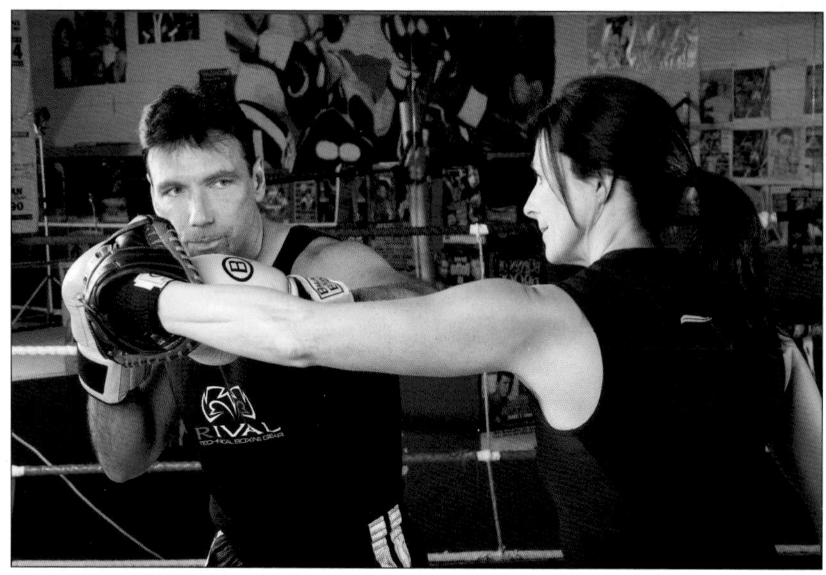

Hook

Combination Three: 1-2/Slip/Right-Left-Right

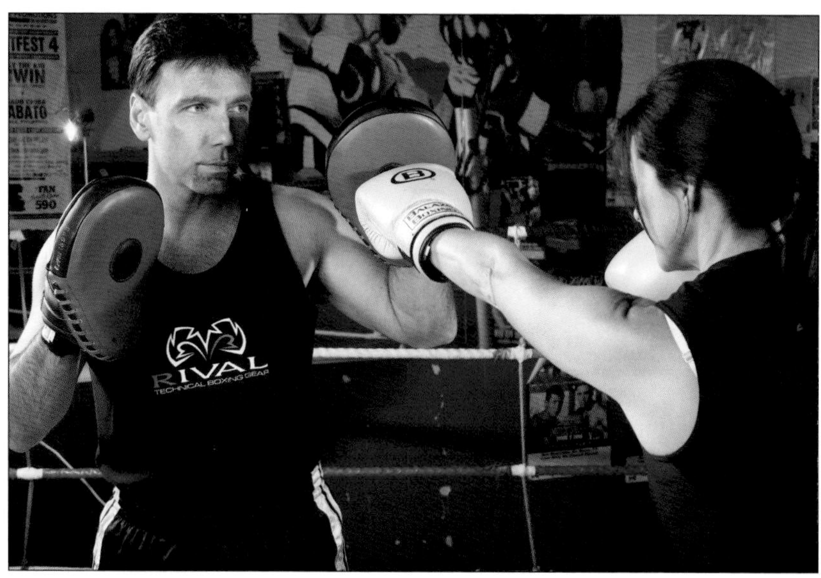

Left jab

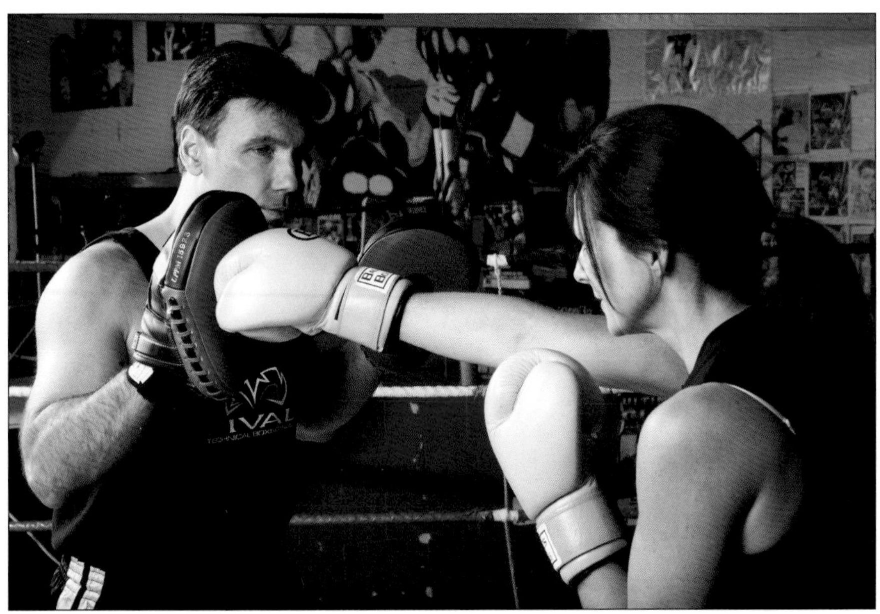

Straight right

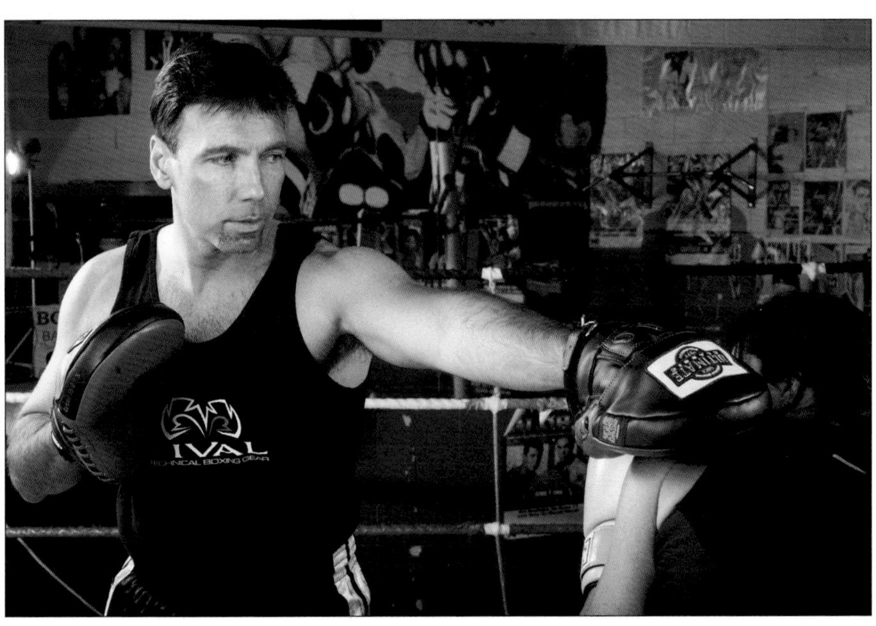

Slip

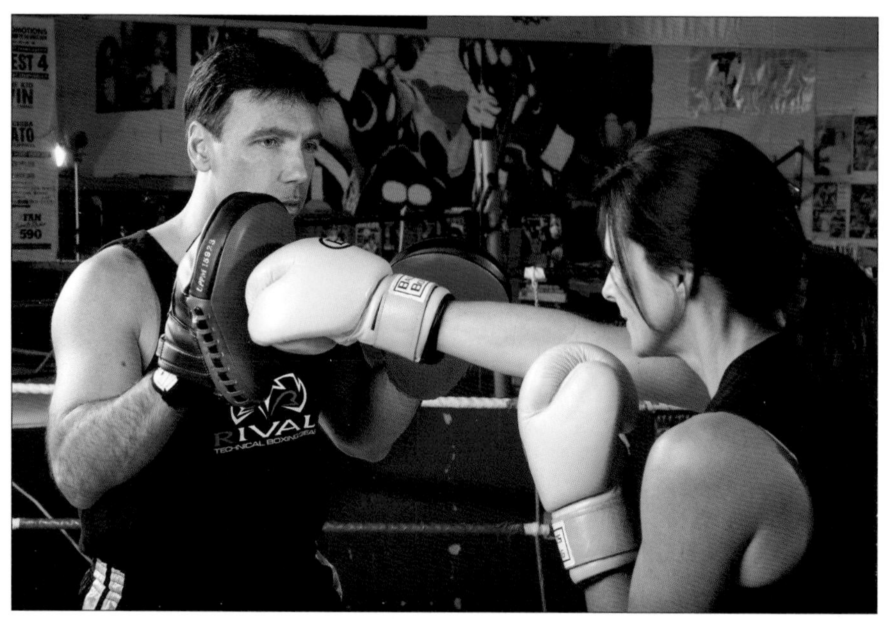

Straight right

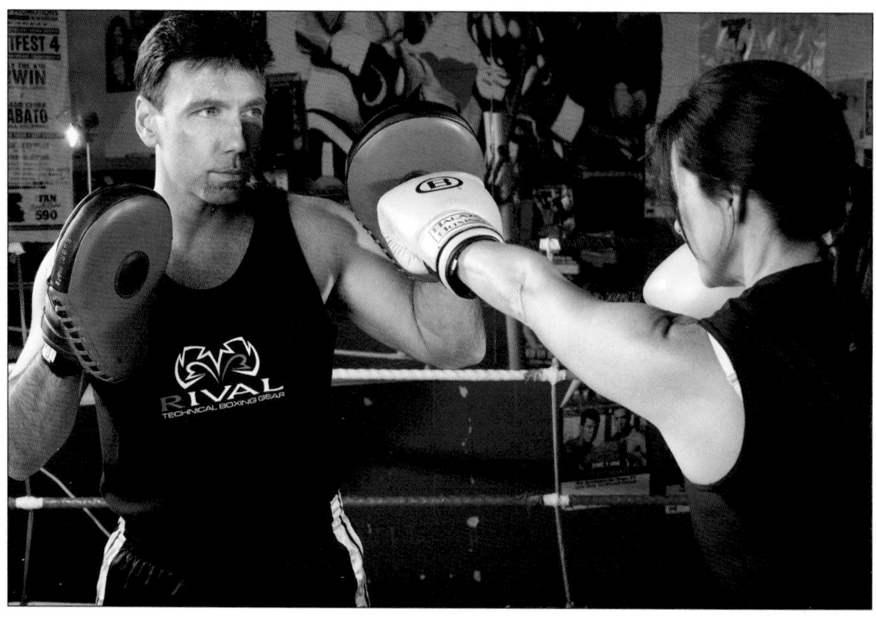

Left jab

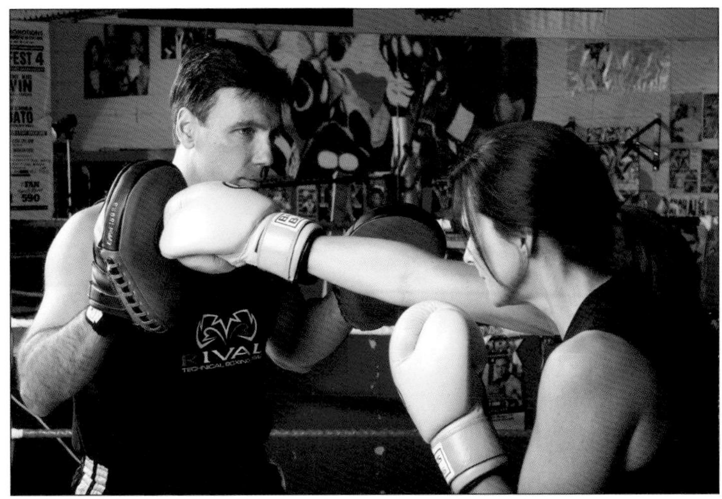

Straight right

Step 1: The puncher starts this drill with a quick 1-2 combination.

Step 2: Catcher throws a left jab as the puncher slips to the right, avoiding the incoming jab.

Step 3: The puncher counters with a right-left-right.

Combination Four: 1-2-1-2/Slip/Slip – Hook/Straight Right

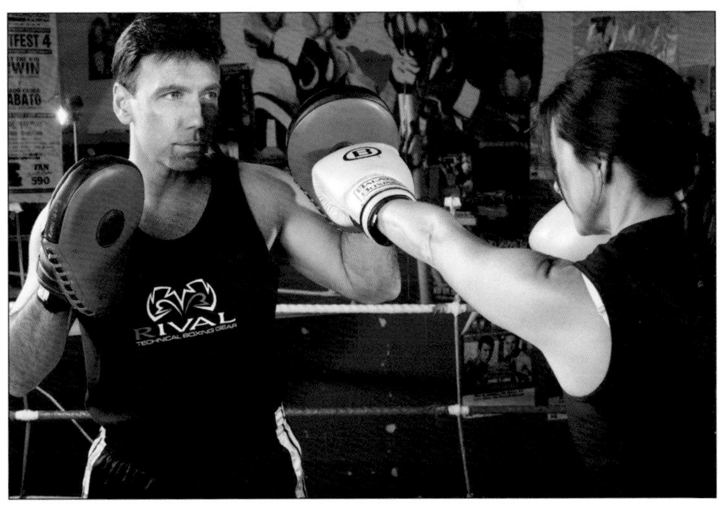

Left jab

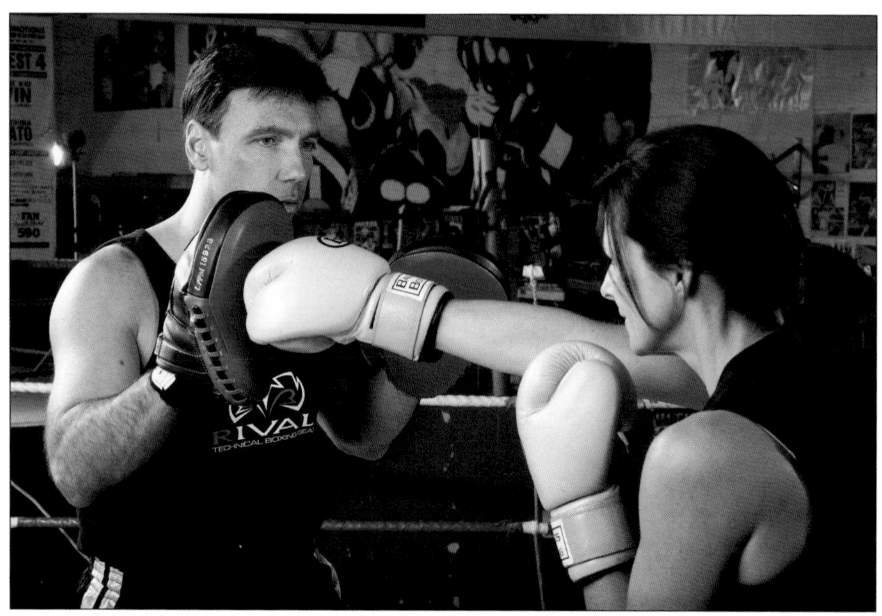

Straight right

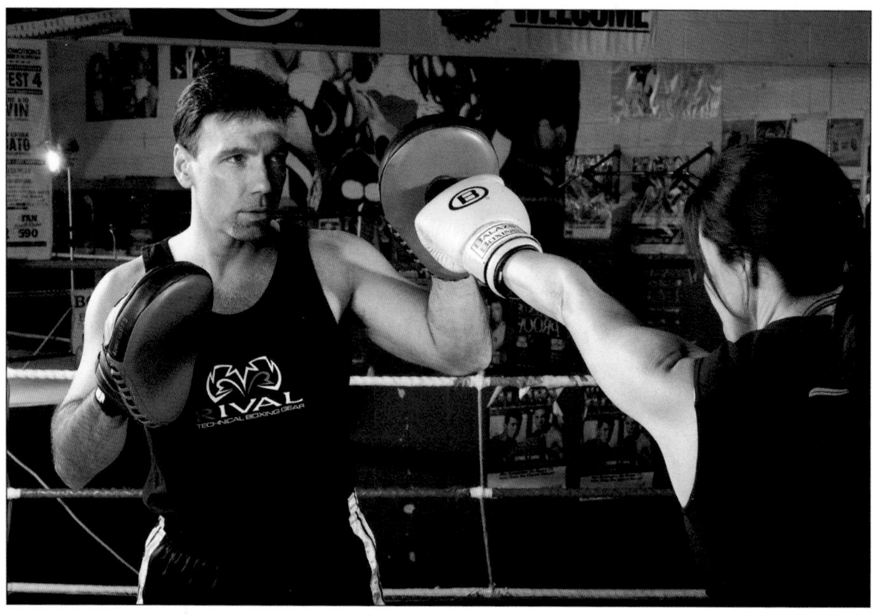

Left jab

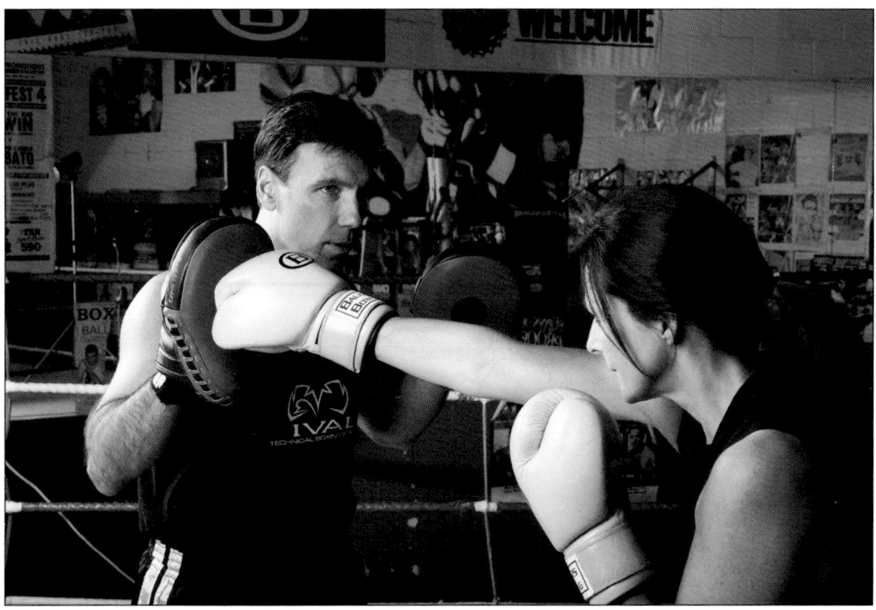

Straight right

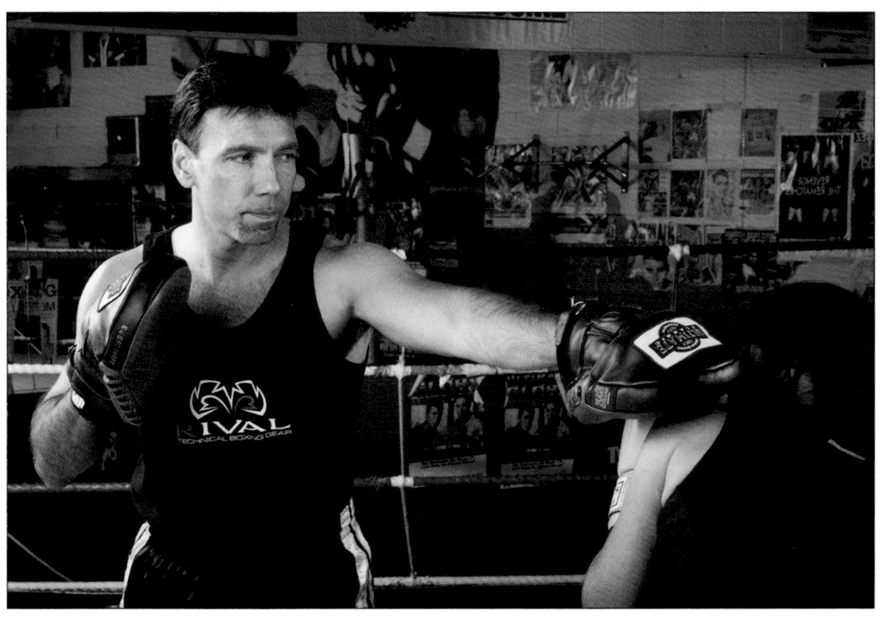

Slip right

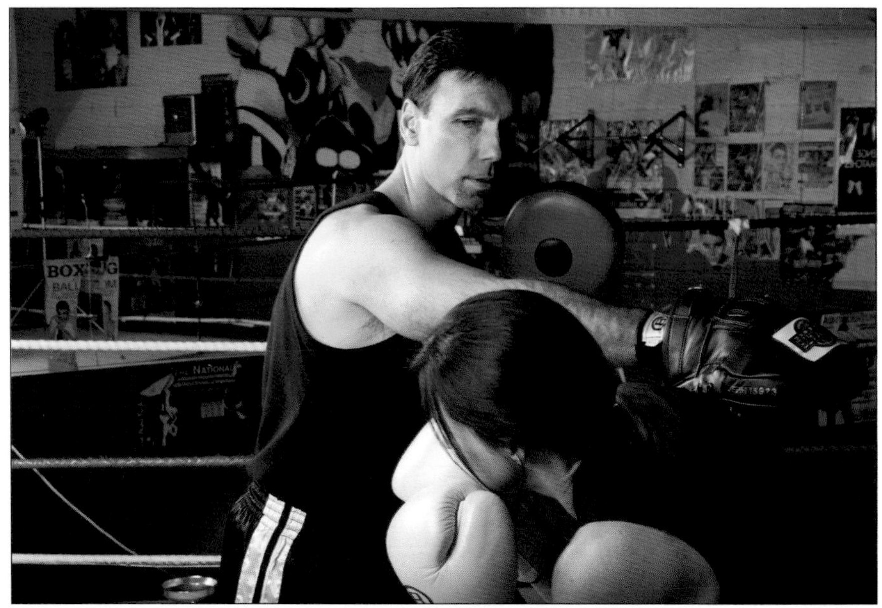

Slip left

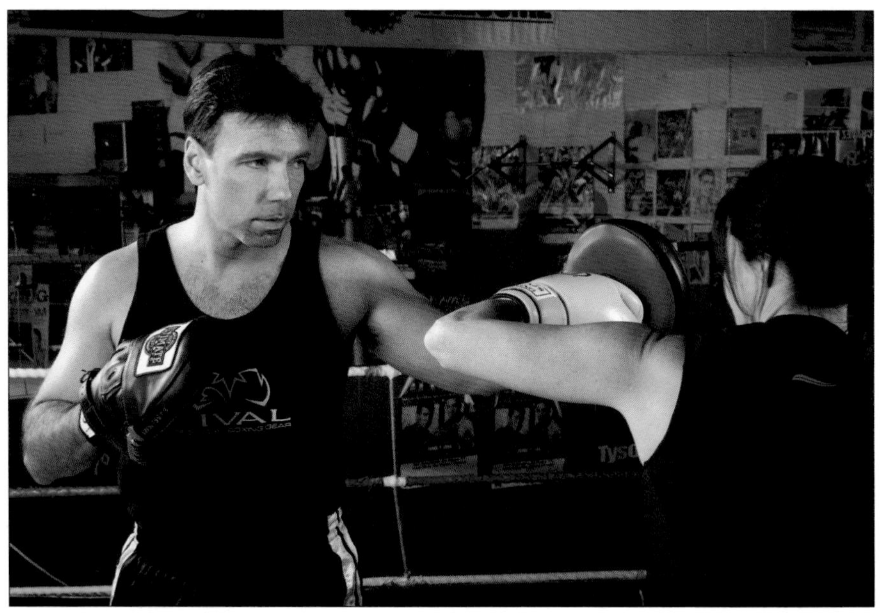

Left hook

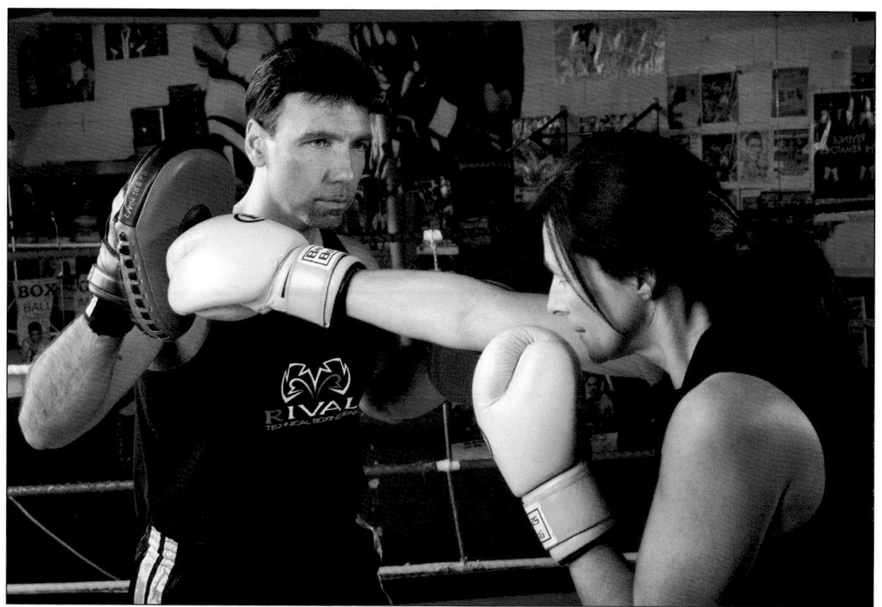

Straight right

Step 1: The puncher throws a 1-2-1-2, slips a left jab and then a straight right.
Step 2: Puncher finishes with a left hook and a straight right.

Combination Five: Uppercut / Uppercut / Uppercut – Left Hook/ Right Cross

Step 1: The catcher prepares to receive three uppercuts. The puncher starts with the right uppercut first, then left, then right.
Step 2: Add a left hook and straight right. This is a quick five-punch combination. It should be smooth and controlled.

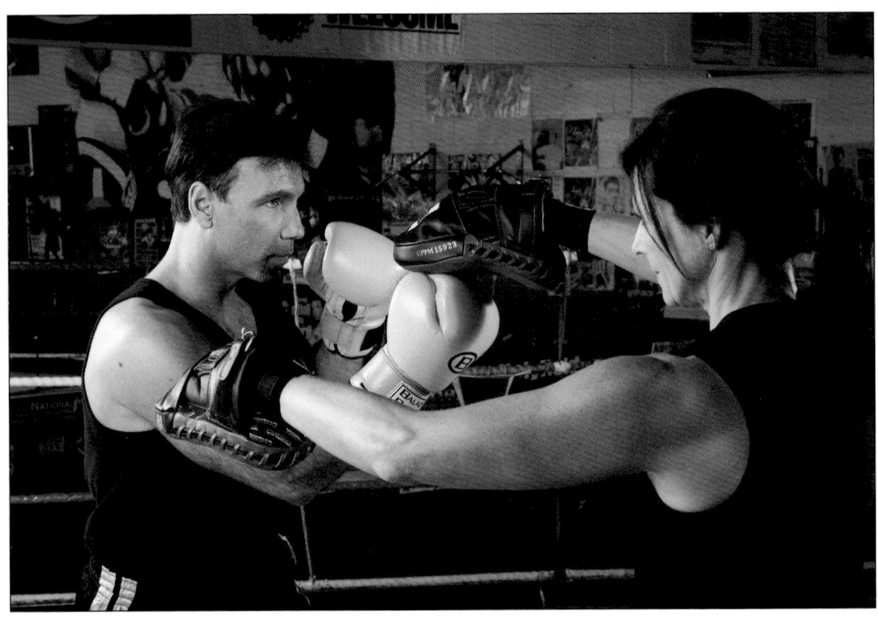

Right uppercut

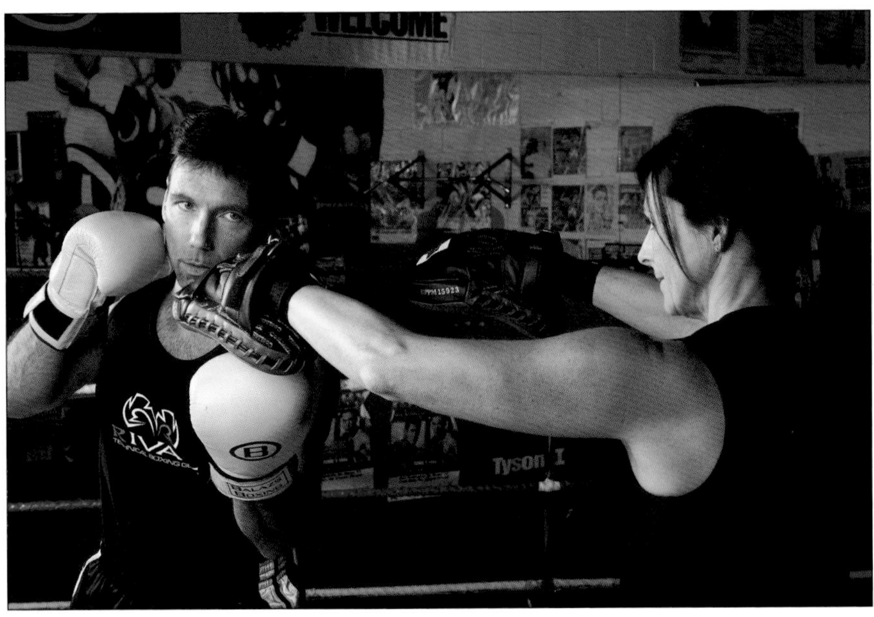

Left uppercut

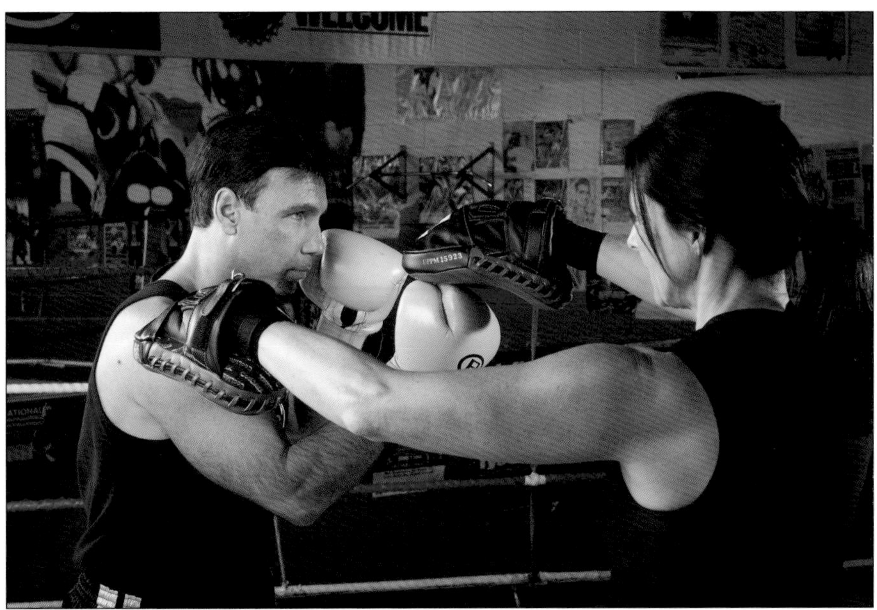

Right uppercut

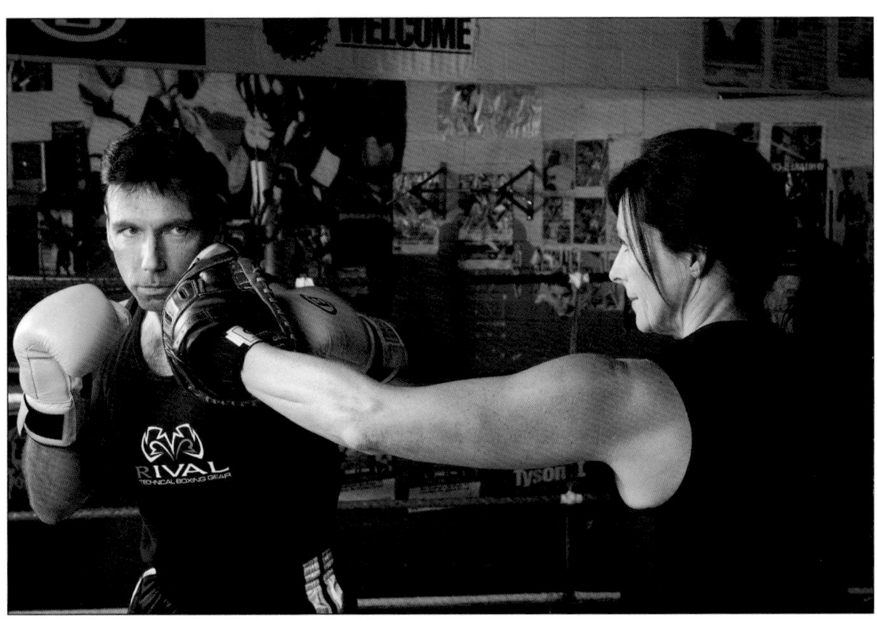

Left Hook

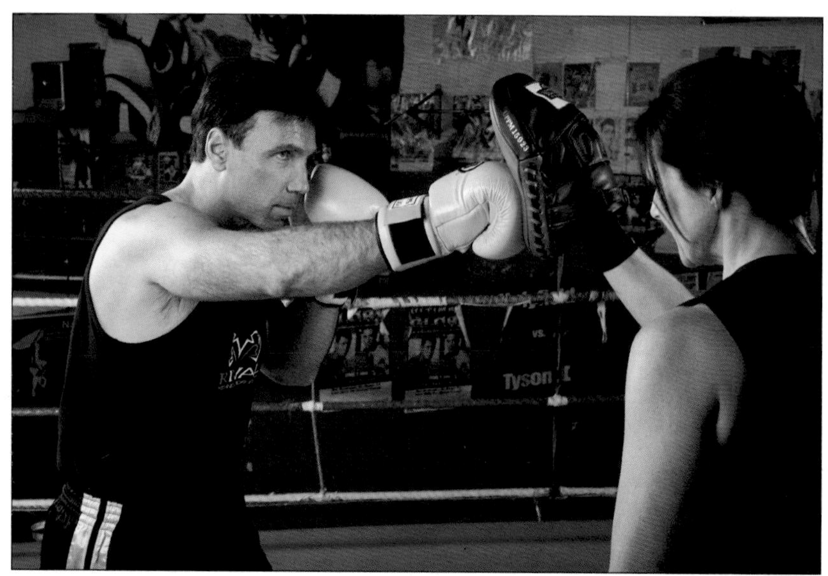

Right cross

Combination Six: Block/Hook/Straight Right – Block – Right/Left/Right

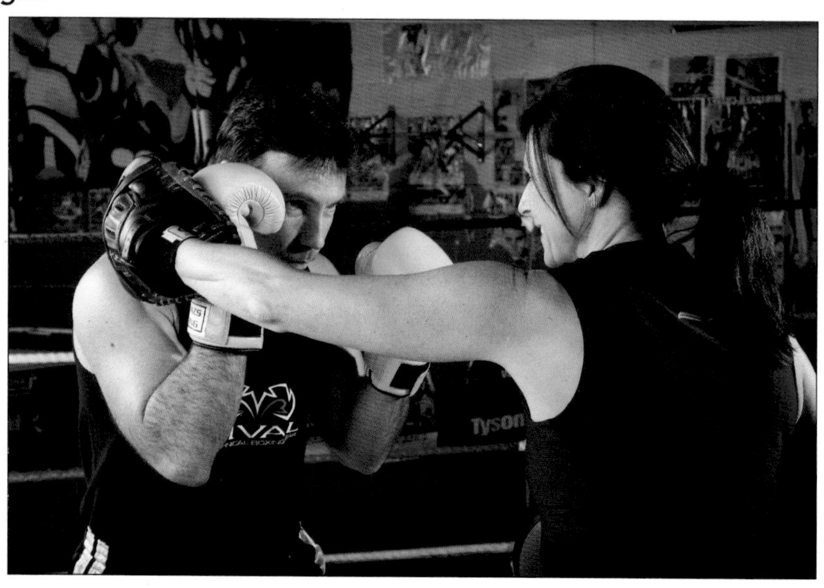

Block

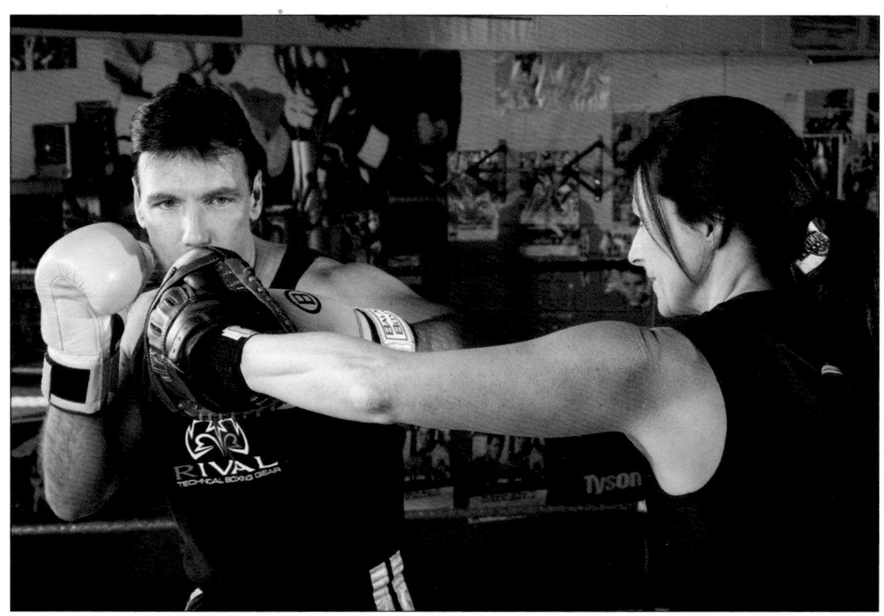

Left hook

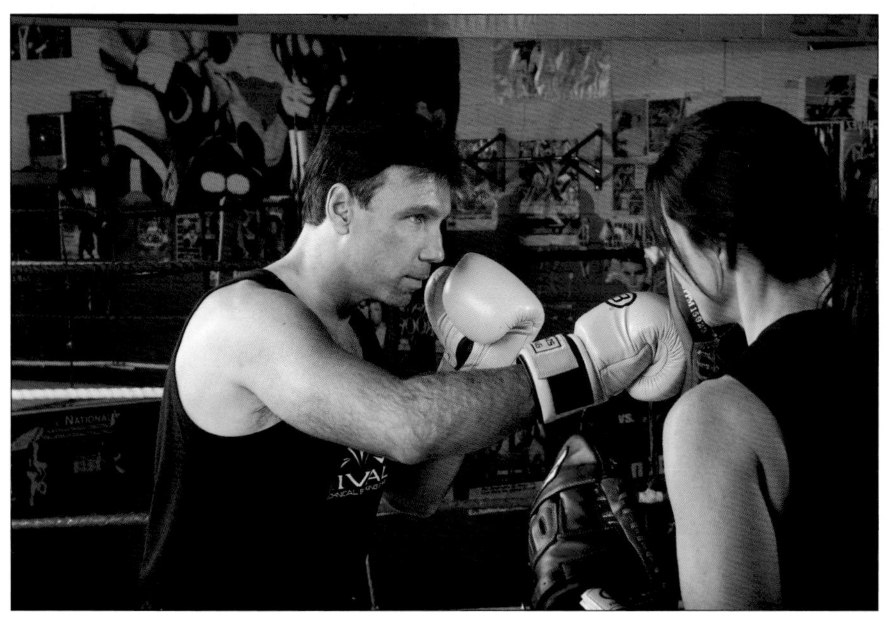

Straight right

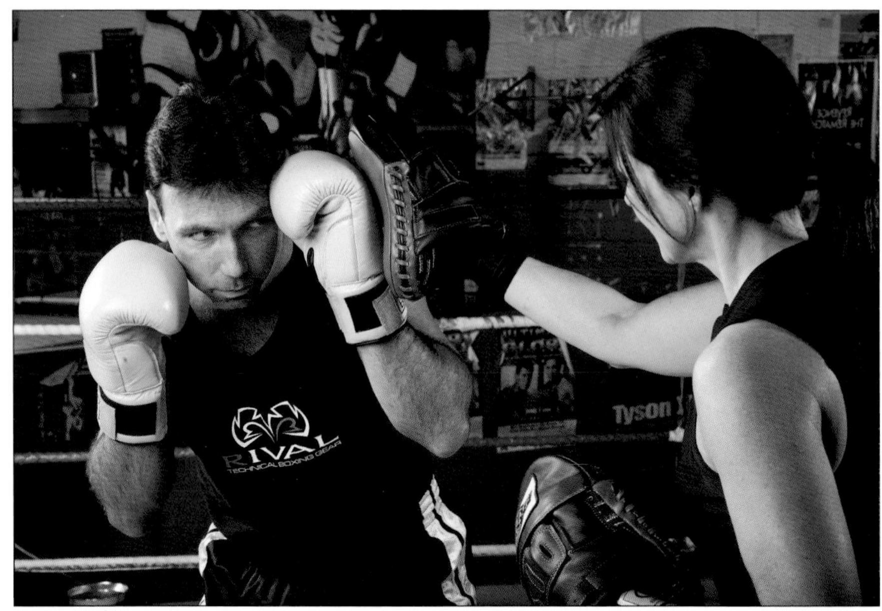

Block

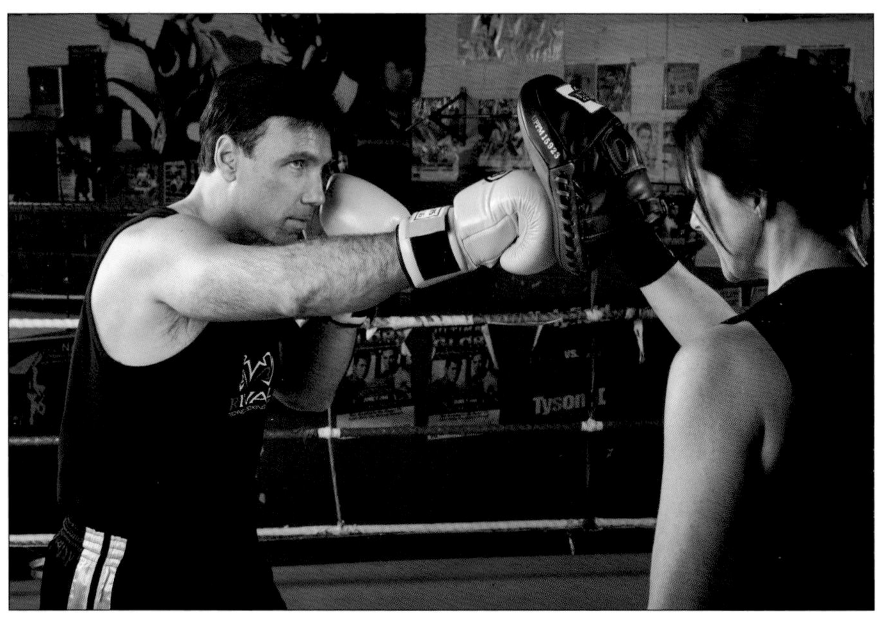

Straight right

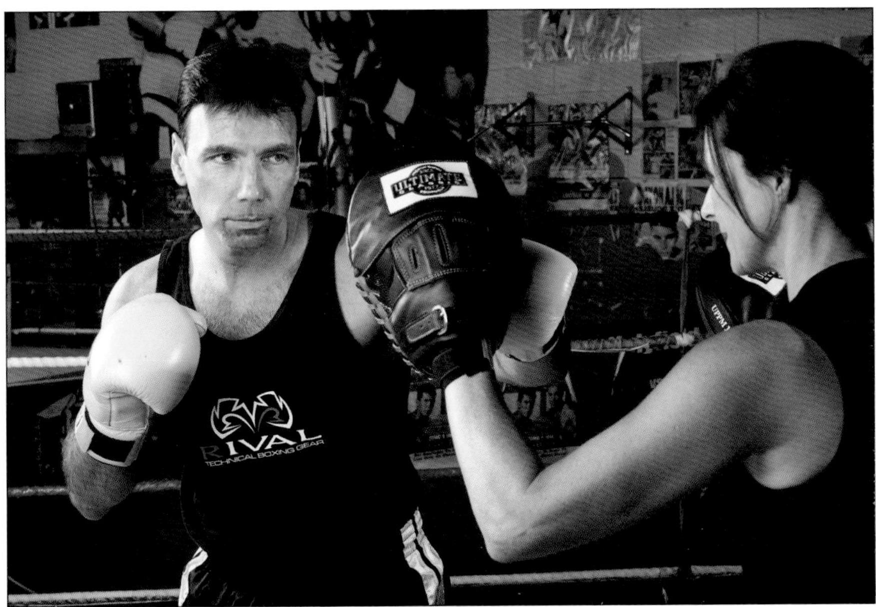

Left jab

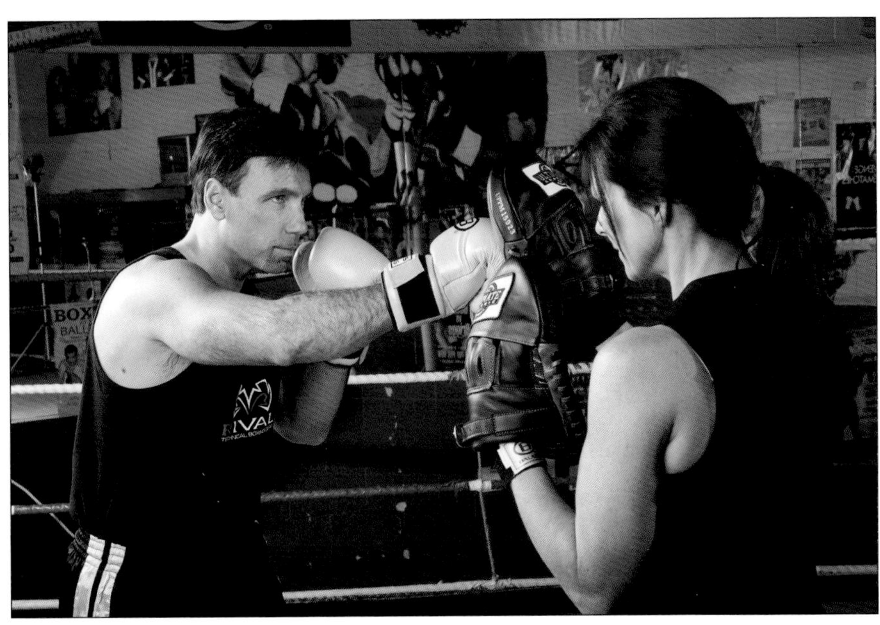

Straight right

Step 1: The puncher holds the hands high in the on-guard position, keeping the gloves tight against the head. The catcher simulates a left hook by lightly tapping the puncher's gloves with the inside (cushion side) of the mitt. The puncher blocks the punch, then fires back with a quick left hook and straight right.
Step 2: The catcher simulates a straight right by lightly tapping the puncher's gloves. The puncher blocks the punch then fires back with a quick straight right, left jab, straight right.

When working punch combinations that require you to slip, block, or parry, move or slip just enough to avoid getting hit.

Target Mitt Sprints

Here is an advanced drill to finish off your boxing workout. This is a speed drill designed to give your muscles one final blast before you cool down.

Catcher

Adjust your target mitts to receive the punches and time the sprint intervals. Have your partner throw his or her straight lefts to your left mitt and straight rights to your right mitt. For the hooks, remember to catch his or her punches with the same hand he or she throws (i.e., catch the right hook with your right hand). For catching uppercuts, you partner should cross over throwing his or her right uppercut to your right target mitt, and so on.

Puncher

Address your partner straight on, with knees bent, leaning slightly forward on the balls of your feet. Get ready to deliver a fast series of punches starting off with straight lefts and rights. Remember to fully extend these punches. You want to go for speed, not power, while maintaining proper form. Without stopping, switch to hooks (left and right) for a short sprint, finishing up with an uppercut sprint.

Sample sprint interval

Straight punches	20 seconds
Hooks	20 seconds
Uppercuts	20 seconds

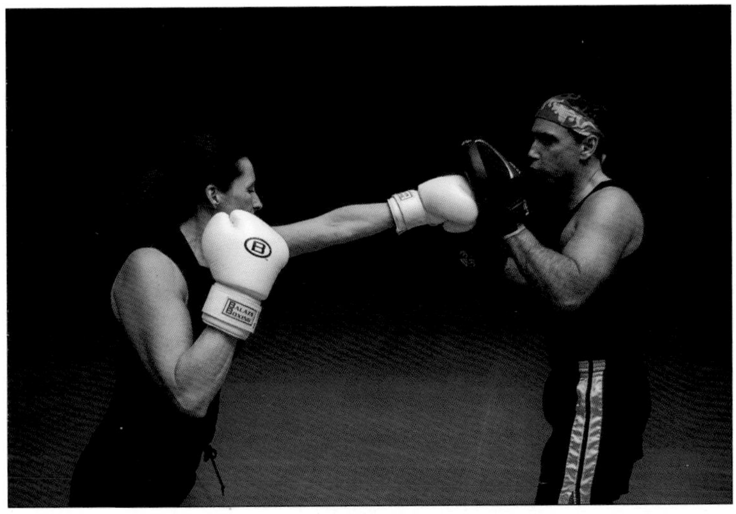

Straight punch

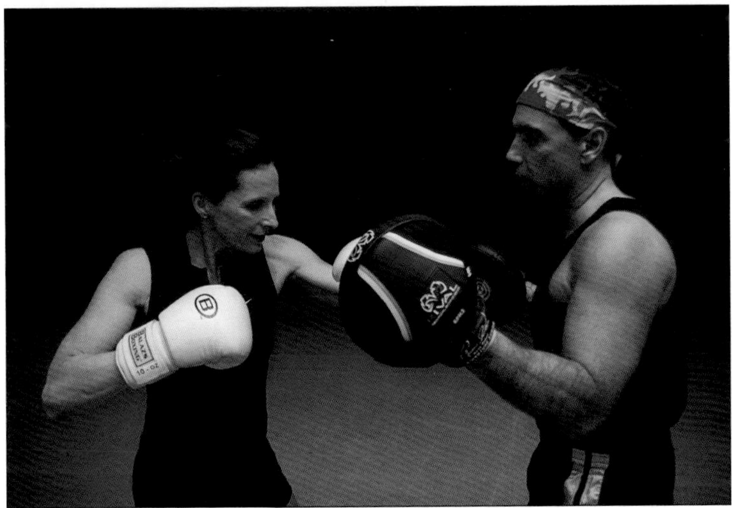

Hook

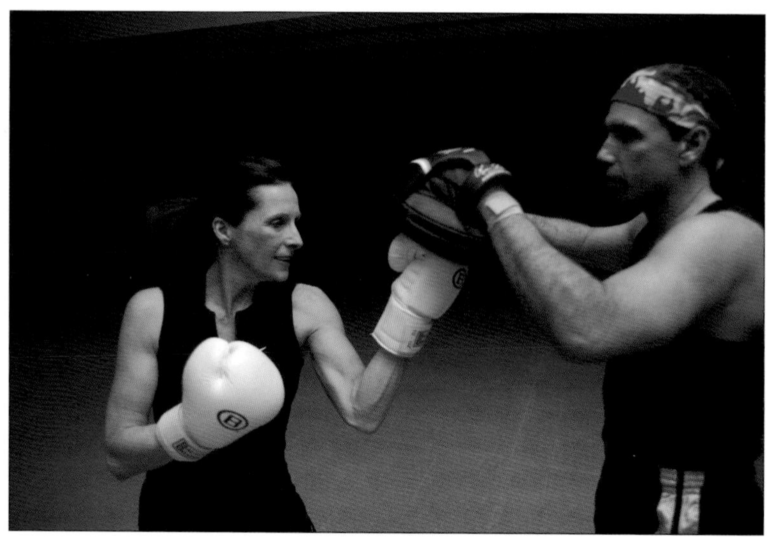

Uppercut

Have your partner go though the sprint sequence twice without a break before you switch partners. Start with twenty-second sprints, eventually working your way up to thirty- or forty-second sprints. This is an advanced drill, so make sure you are thoroughly warmed up.

Learning the Ropes

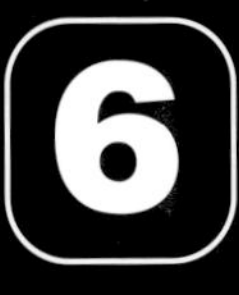

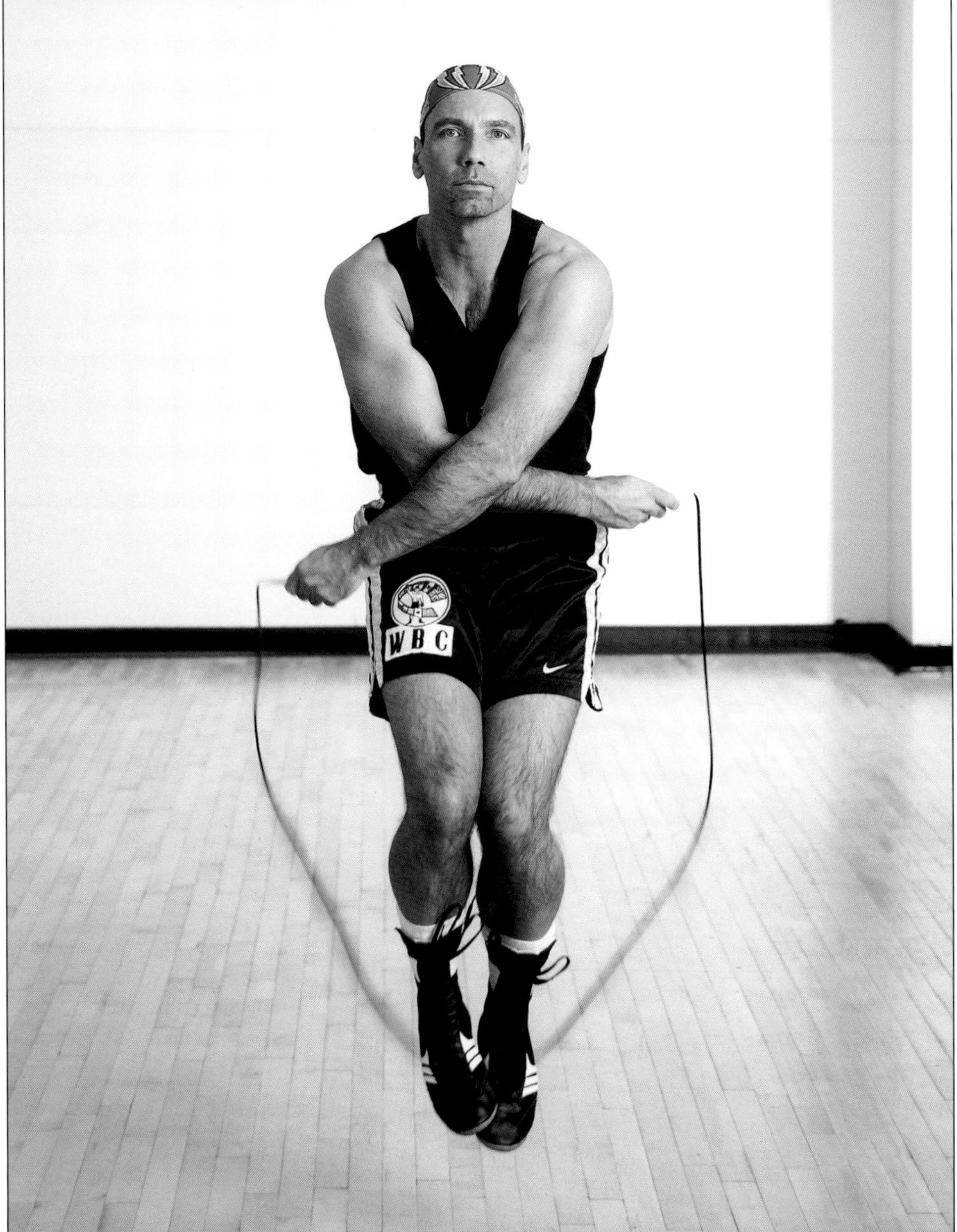

Learning the Ropes

Jump rope is one of the single best exercises you can engage in. In just fifteen to twenty minutes, jump rope will give you an unparalleled total body workout. Not only will jumping rope improve your cardiovascular endurance, it will also lead to significant gains in your performance level for virtually any sport—baseball, football, skiing, basketball, tennis, volleyball, and more. Eye-hand-foot coordination is trained, improving agility and fluidity, lateral movement, explosiveness, hand and foot speed, and timing. Jumping rope will help you "float like a butterfly and sting like a bee."

The greatest boxer of all time, Muhammad Ali, would dazzle his opponents with his fancy footwork and then throw a barrage of lightning-fast punches. Ali would dance around the ring and shuffle, rapidly alternating his feet front and back. If you ever had the opportunity to watch him shuffling his feet while jumping rope, keeping time, moving smoothly, you understand how he was so successful when he danced across the canvas during a fight.

Jumping rope requires a level of discipline not found in other aerobic activities. It is important to stay focused and in control, all the while concentrating on the feet, balance, and timing. It takes some time and commitment to master the basic jumps, but once this is accomplished, a wide variety of combinations can be performed. This not only makes the workout fun, it also challenges a large variety of muscles. It works the gluteals, quadriceps, calves, and hamstrings. The upper body, the back and chest muscles, deltoids, forearms, biceps, and triceps are recruited to produce the movement of rotating and stabilizing the rope. To maintain proper alignment and the correct center of gravity, the abdominal muscles are recruited to contract and hold the body position. Jumping rope challenges the cardiovascular system and improves coordination, which in turn helps to develop boxing agility, timing, power, and speed. It's a great total-body workout to improve overall conditioning.

Jumping rope is something that can be taught to virtually anyone and can be learned within weeks of starting, even though it can be demanding and at the very least frustrating when starting out. Many think that it is just too difficult to learn, and that a cardiovascular workout will not be accomplished because they will not be able to keep jumping for twenty minutes. A teaching method based on neutral and resting moves and a three-step breakdown is used successfully in fifteen and twenty minute jump rope classes and allows even the novice to feel triumphant. People also think that skipping is simply boring and too repetitive. But there is a lot more to it than just jumping up and down

Neutral and resting moves are incorporated in the jumping because it is difficult, and sometimes feels impossible, for beginners to continuously jump through (or inside) a rope for more than a few minutes at a time before stopping. In fact, it can be a humbling experience for even the best-conditioned athlete. Instead of stopping and just putting your rope down when you feel that you just can't continue jumping, put both handles in one hand and continue to perform the jump with the rope turning to the side of the body. At this point you are jumping "outside" the rope. A basic jog or march while continually turning the rope can keep the heart rate elevated and may reduce the frustration of stopping and starting. Accomplished jump ropers use neutral or resting moves to add variety to their cardio workout allowing for higher and lower training intensities.

The Three-Step Breakdown divides up more complicated moves into manageable moves that can be easily practiced and learned. This systematic training method starts with the footwork being practiced without the rope. In the second step, both handles of the rope are placed into one hand, and the new move is executed while turning the rope at one side, much like the neutral or resting moves. The third step is performing the move inside of the rope. Whenever you have a more challenging foot pattern that you want to perform, the three-step breakdown will help you succeed.

Three-Step Breakdown

Step 1: Practice the foot and arm movements without the rope to give yourself a feel for the moves and the timing.
Step 2: Continue the movement and add the rope (both handles in one hand), turning it to the side of the body (a neutral and resting move).
Step 3: Continue the movement and now jump through the rope.

Equipment

There are a variety of ropes to choose from: Plastic, beaded, and leather. A rope that is too long or too short will force you to adjust the position of the arms, causing poor execution of movement and jumping technique. A plastic segmented or "beaded" jump rope, weighing about half a pound allows for the length to be adjusted, customizing it specifically for the height required. A rope that is too light will not hold a true arc, and it will become more easily tangled and not be able to create a sufficient amount of momentum to produce the desired motion. Conversely, a rope that is too heavy produces slow, cumbersome rotations, increases the risk of injury at the wrists and shoulders, and increases pain on impact when you miss. Look for a rope that has comfortable, durable, and well-constructed handles, perhaps covered in a foam material to help reduce the handle movement in your hands.

Form and Technique: How to Jump

Start with proper form and good technique. Whether you are just starting to jump or performing an array of masterful foot and arm movements, there are a few rules to follow:

- Jump only an inch or two off of the ground.
- Keep the knees slightly bent.

- Land softly on the ground, rolling through the balls of the feet in order for the legs to absorb the impact.
- Keep the jumps in control with the torso upright. Do not allow the body to lean forward or backward.
- Initiate the action of the turning of the rope at the wrist, with little movement at the shoulders or arms (a proper weight of rope will assist in reduced shoulder and arm movement).
- Keep the shoulders down and relaxed.
- Keep the arms at one level and upper part of the arm close to the sides of the body. Be careful not to allow the arms to drift away from the body because this will raise the rope higher from the floor and closer to the jumping feet, resulting in the rope becoming entangled in the feet.
- Keep the head in a neutral position and the neck relaxed.

It does take practice, and practice pays off. Within a few weeks, you will be putting together foot and arms combinations that will improve your agility, balance, and cardiovascular abilities.

The best surface to jump on is a wood-sprung floor at a gym because it reduces stress on the legs and feet. Or if there is a ring around, jump in it.

Executing a Neutral Move

One of the more difficult challenges in jumping rope is to keep going, and as previously mentioned, the neutral move helps you through wanting to just throw the rope down and quit. Keep the feet moving, jump up and down, and place both handles in one hand. The body, shoulders, arms, and wrists should be in the proper position as the rope turns at the side of the body. Try not to let the rope wander in front of the body. Change the rope to the other hand once in a while to add variety, and to get comfortable with different arm positions.

Jumps and Combinations

The Basic Two-Foot Jump

(Difficulty level 1)

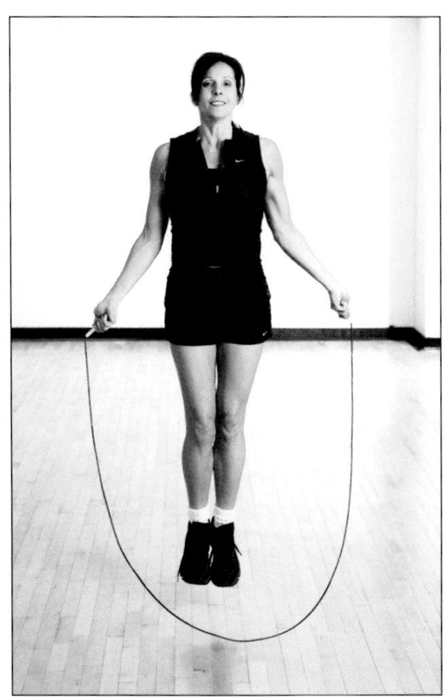

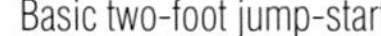

Basic two-foot jump-start

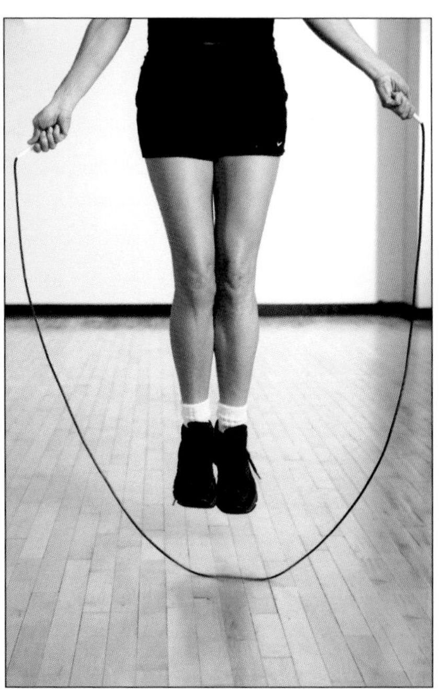

Basic two-foot jump-finish

Stand on the floor with the rope behind the feet and both feet side by side. Relax the head and shoulders, and keep the head straight forward. Keep the arms by the side of the body, with the hands holding onto the rope comfortably. Push off of the floor with the feet, jumping into the air while rotating the rope upward behind the back, over the head, in front of the body, and under the feet. Remember the arms stay by the side of the body and rotate the rope with the wrists. The handles of the rope stay the same distance away from the floor. The feet come only an inch to an inch and a half inch off of the floor (avoid jumping too high or kicking the feet back). Land on the balls of the feet, rolling through them, and keep the knees slightly bent in order to absorb part of the impact. Repeat, varying the speed to change intensity levels.

Boxer's Skip

(Difficulty level 1)

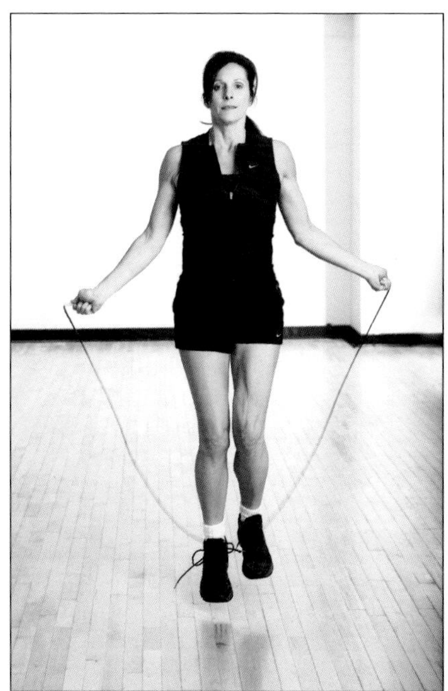

Boxer's skip

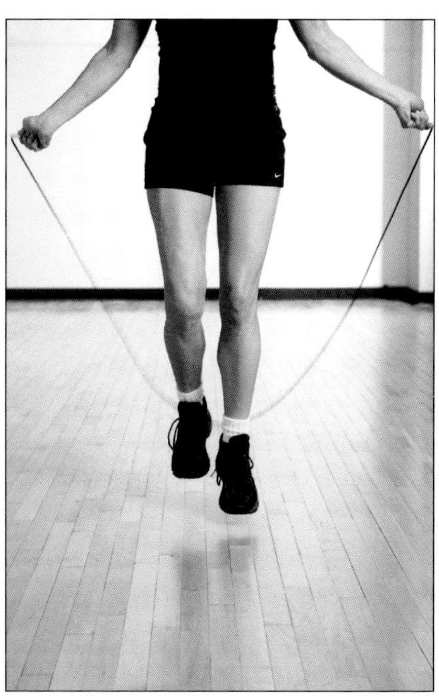

Boxer's skip close-up

Start with the basic two-skip jump and shift your weight from one foot to the other. Keep the knees slightly bent, and push off from one foot at a time. The feet stay close to the floor as in the basic two-foot jump. Relax the shoulders and neck. Obtain a rhythm from side to side, varying the footwork slightly. Example: Right foot, left foot, two rights. Then, left foot, right foot, two lefts. Repeat and add in the basic two-foot jump.

Ski Jump

(Difficulty level 2)

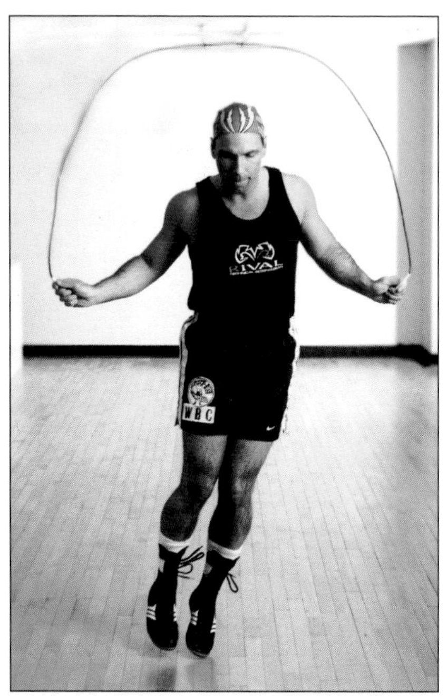

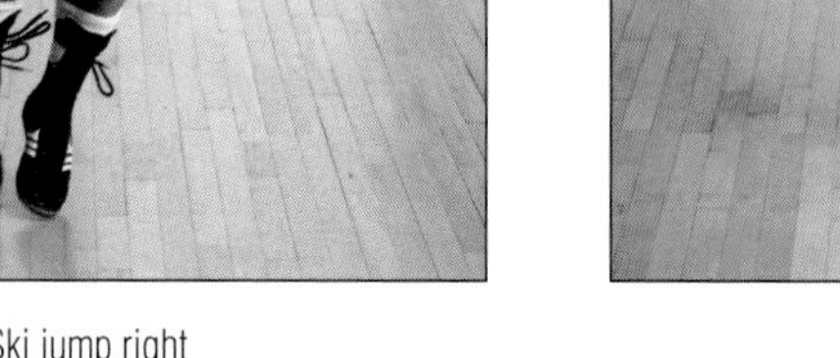

Ski jump right

Ski jump left

Perform the basic two-foot jump while landing to the right side of your starting point and then the left side. When learning this jump, it sometimes helps to jump to one side, jump back to the center, then jump to the other side, then back to the center. Repeat until you feel comfortable, then take out the center jump. Remember to keep the arms by the side of the body and to rotate the rope at the wrists. With the addition of the side-to-side or front-to-back movement, the arms have a tendency to travel outward, which will result in the rope becoming entangled in the feet. Stay relaxed through the shoulder and neck areas and find your rhythm.

One-Foot Kicks

(Difficulty level 2)

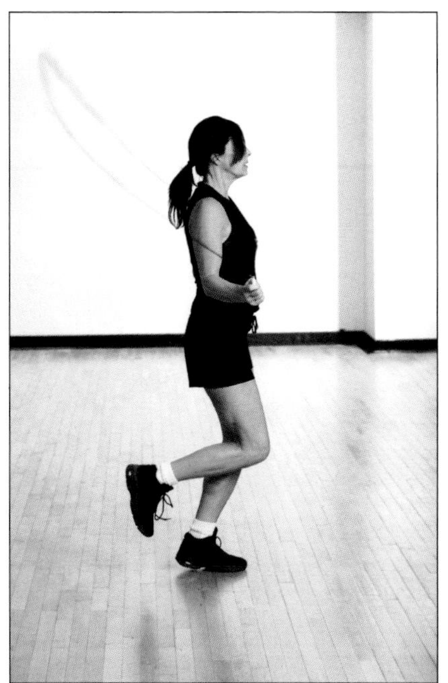

One-foot kick-start

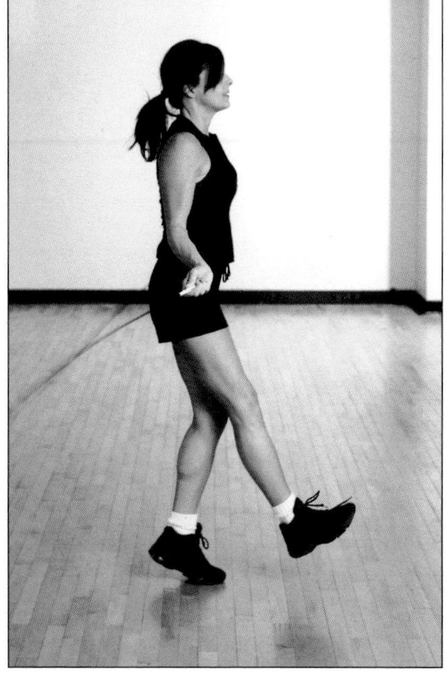

One-foot kick-finish

Start with the basic two-foot jump. Jump on the floor with one foot, kicking the other foot back and then kicking it forward. Perform a basic two-foot jump again and repeat the kick with the other foot. Then a basic two-foot jump. Try to increase difficulty by traveling forward and backward and by lifting the kicking leg higher.

High Knees

(Difficulty level 3)

Start with the boxer's skip, and lift the knees higher in front. Ensure that you land softly, a slight bend at the knee. Keep the body upright, arms and

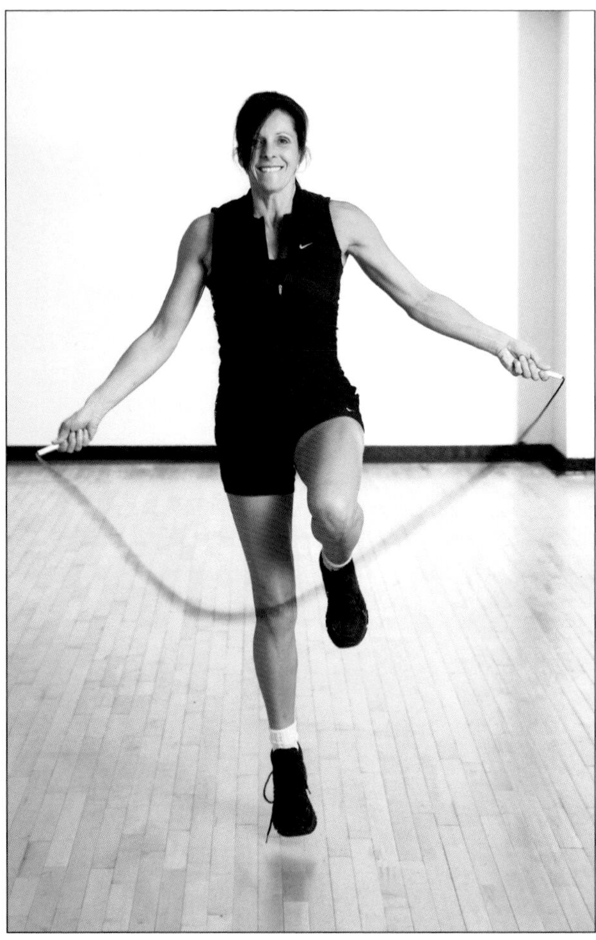

High knees

hands in the proper position. Focus on the push-off phase of one foot and then the other, lifting the knees as high as possible. By practicing this jump, you will help improve the muscle power in each ankle and leg. Try performing ten to twenty high knees. Then go back to the boxer's skip to recover. You may also want to add direction into the jump by traveling forward for eight jumps and backward for eight jumps.

Jumping Jacks /Stride Jumps

(Difficulty level 3)

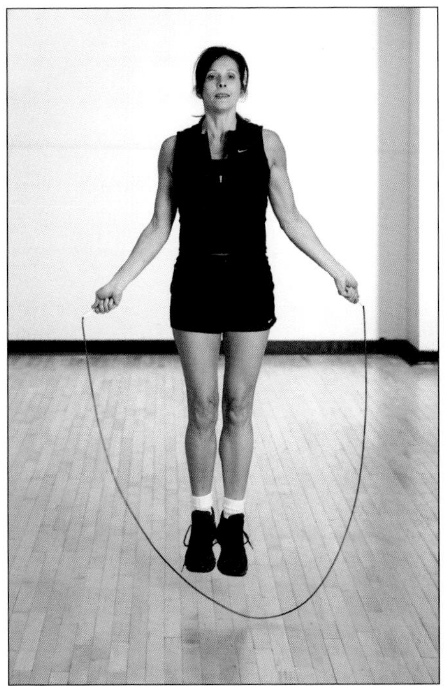

Jumping jacks-start

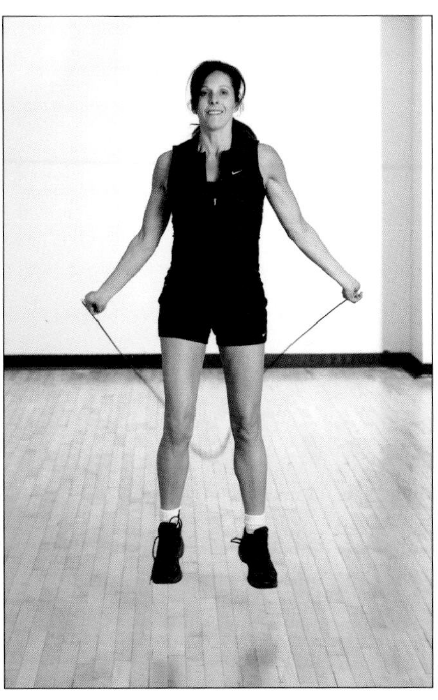

Jumping jacks-finish

Start with a basic two-foot jump, and jump, separating the feet about shoulder-width. Land with the feet in this position, push off again, and bring the feet back together in the air before landing on the floor with the feet together. When performing this jump, be careful not to make the foot separation too wide because the rope will most likely get tangled with your feet. The longer the rope, the farther the feet can be separated.

Ali Shuffle

(Difficulty level 3)

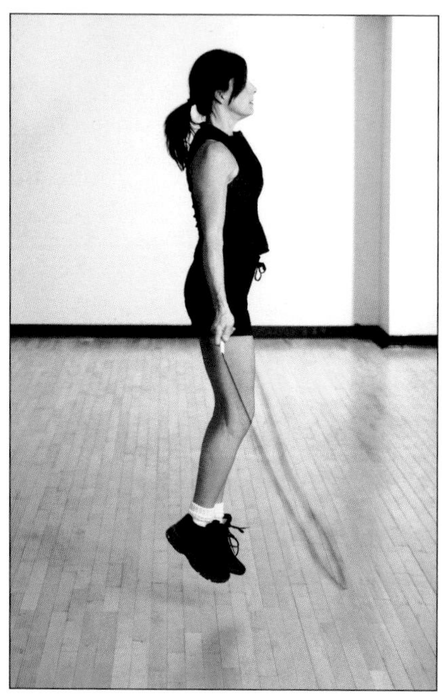

Ali shuffle–start

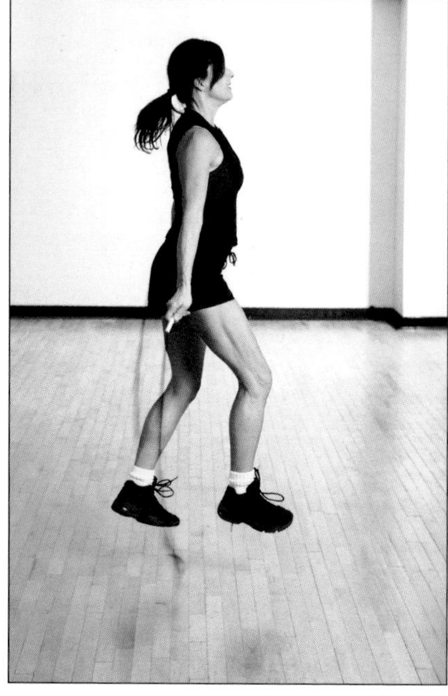

Ali shuffle–finish

This is the boxer's jump, with the addition of moving the feet front and back. As you jump in the air, move one foot forward slightly and one foot backward slightly, and then land with both on the floor. Push off of the floor again, taking the front foot towards the back and the back foot towards the front, landing with both feet on the floor. Repeat, landing softly and moving quickly. The center of gravity changes slightly as one foot is in front and the other is in back, challenging your agility and response time. Muhammad Ali was known for his quick foot movements, shuffling across the canvas from side to side and frustrating his opponents. Practicing this jump will teach you to be on your toes, moving and changing your foot positioning and maintaining a center of balance, ready for any directional change.

Scissors

(Difficulty level 4)

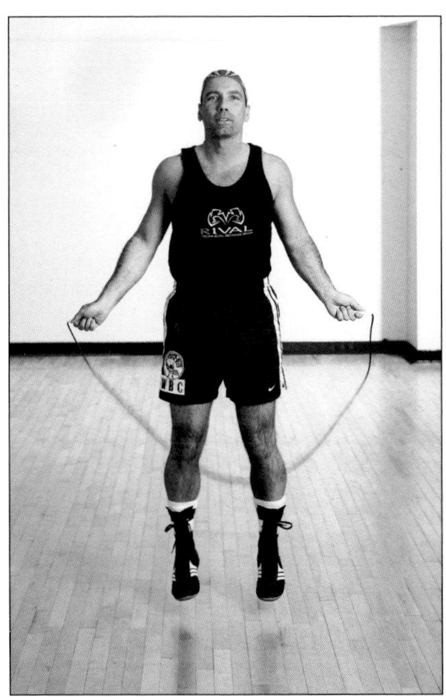

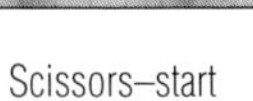

Scissors–start

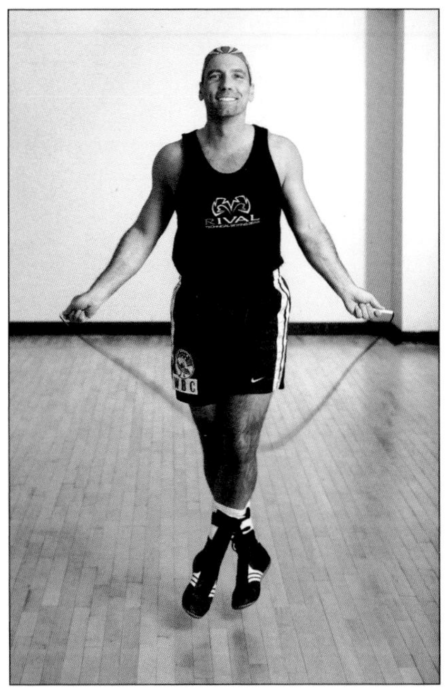

Scissors–finish

Similar to the stride jump, start with the basic two-foot jump, and jump separating the feet to about shoulder width, land, and push off again. Cross the legs while in the air, and land with the feet crossed. Push off, landing with the feet shoulder-width apart. Push off and cross the legs again, landing with the other foot crossed in front.

Ali Shuffle and Jumping Jacks

(Difficulty level 4)

To improve agility, timing, and balance, combine the Ali shuffle with jumping jacks. Start with eight shuffles, then eight jacks. Reduce down to shuffle and a single jack. Shuffle-shuffle-jack.

Diamond Jump

(Difficulty level 4)

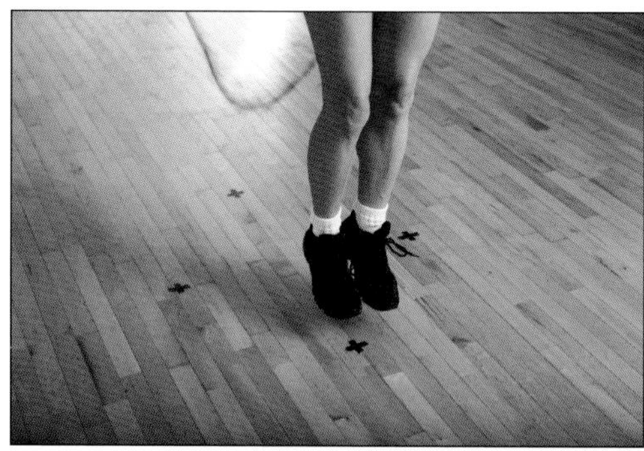

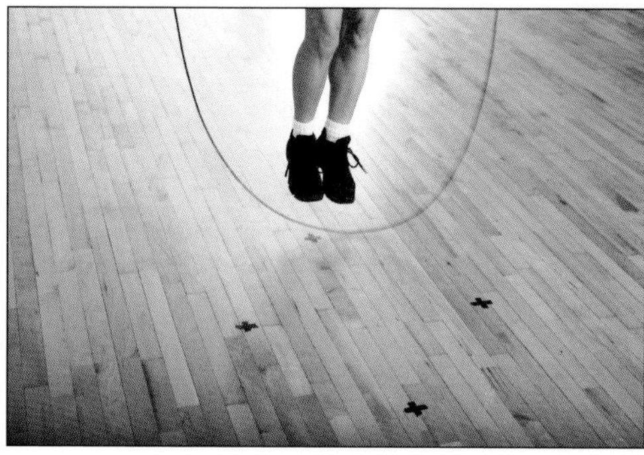

Taking the basic two-foot jump, push off with both feet, moving six to eight inches to a point on the diamond. Because a single jump is performed at each point of the diamond, this is a great test for agility and leg power. Then change direction and repeat the jumps. Return to the boxer's skip when tired.

Double Jumps

(Difficulty level 5)

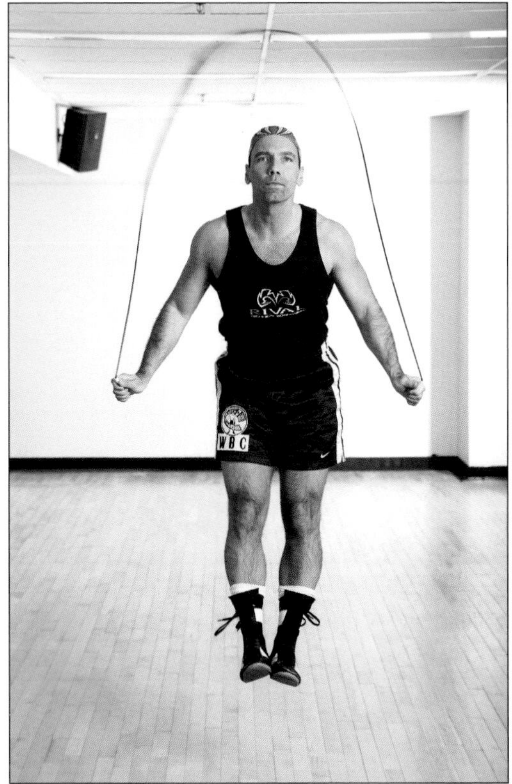

Double jump

This jump will deposit you right into anaerobic land. Two rotations of the rope, one magnified jump! To perform this jump, the rope speed must be faster, and the jump must be substantially higher than the basic jump. This is one jump that challenges both muscular strength and cardiovascular fitness. To start, perform four to six double jumps before going back to the basic two-foot jumps. Repeat, trying to reduce the number of basic jumps performed between the double jumps. For a real blast, work, up to three sets of twenty double jumps with the basic two-foot skip or boxer's skip in between the sets.

Crossovers

(Difficulty level 5)

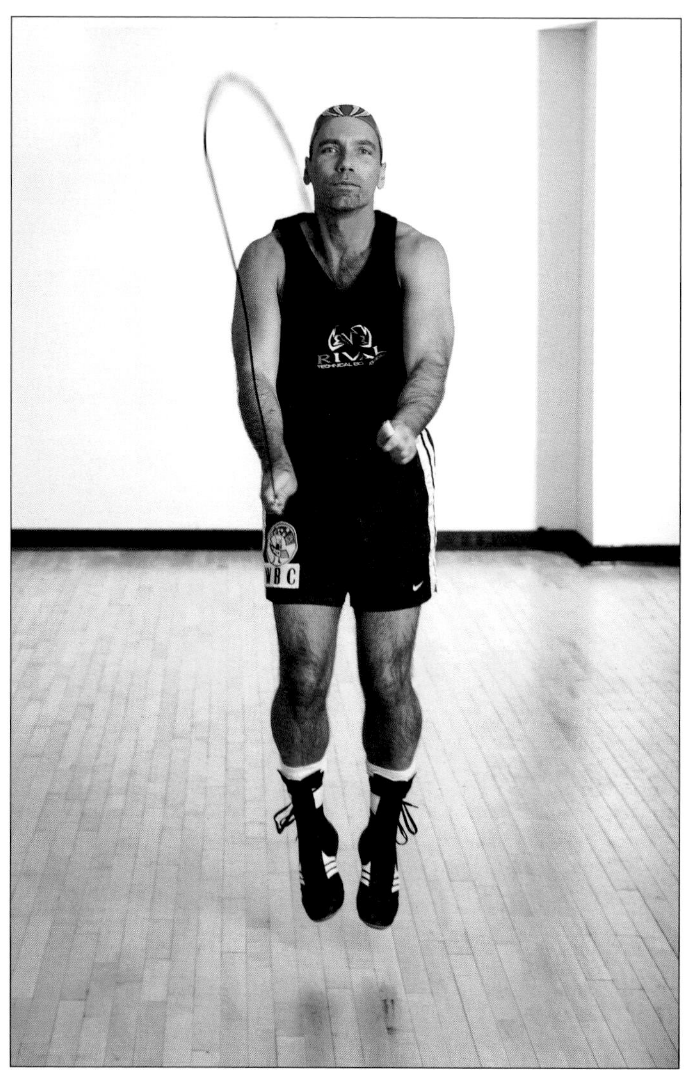

Crossover–start

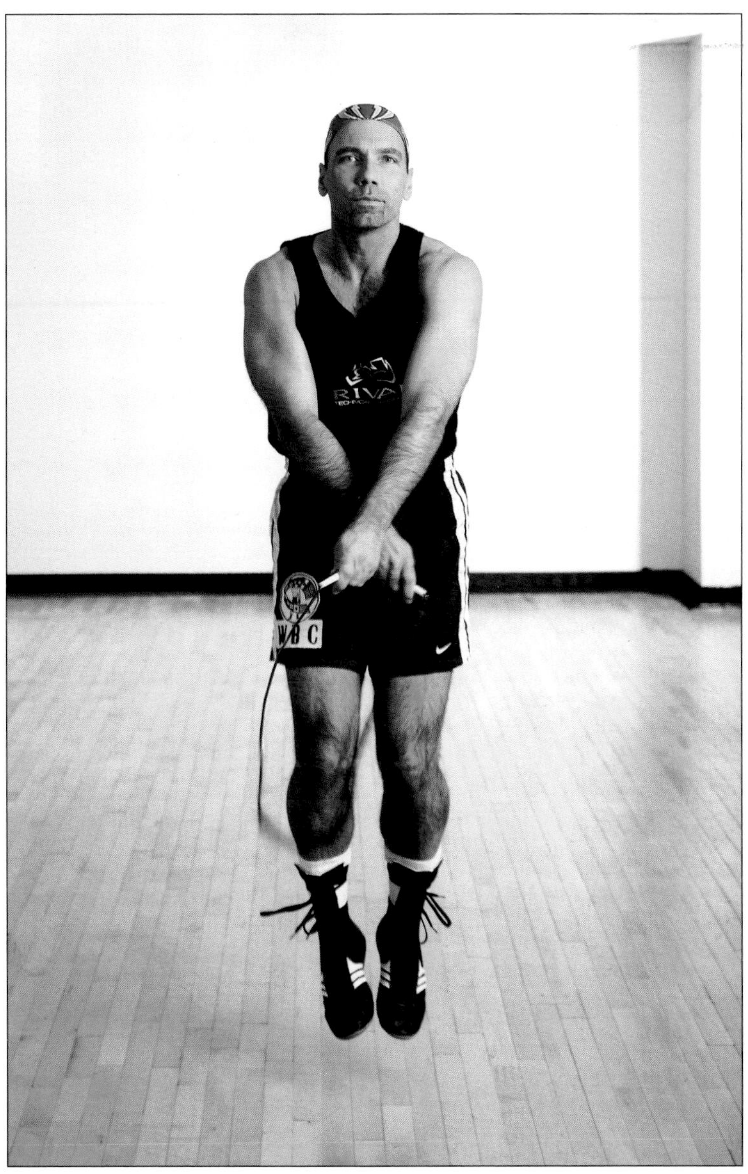

Cross arms

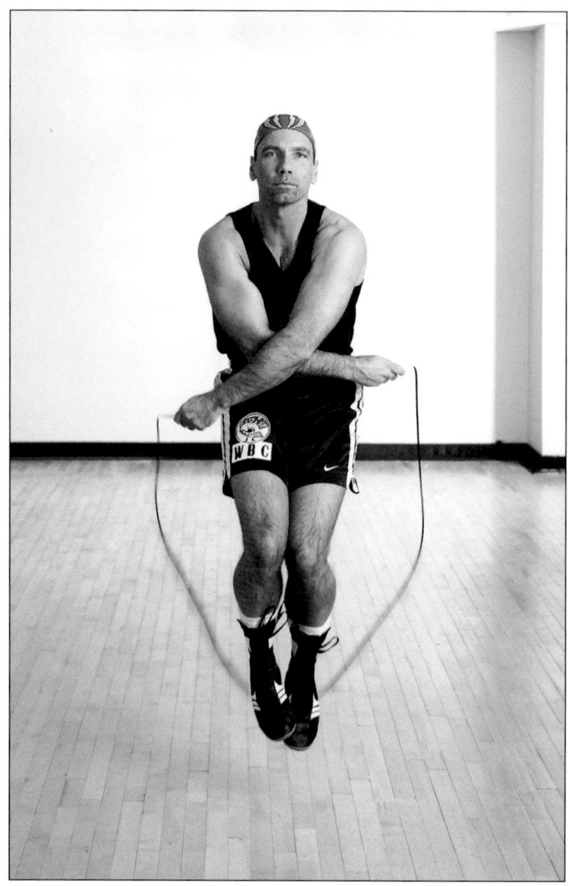

Crossover–finish

Start with the basic two-foot jump. When the rope is overhead, cross the arms at waist level. The left hand will be at the right hip, and the right hand will be at the left hip. Keep the wrists straight and the rope handles pointing out to the sides, not downwards. As the rope comes down towards the toes, jump over it. And as it comes overhead again, uncross the arms. The hands will be at the starting position now. Perform a few basic jumps and repeat the crossovers. With just a little practice, crossover jumps can be repeated many times in a row, traveling forward, backward, and in a circle.

Figure-Eight Jump

(Difficulty level 5)

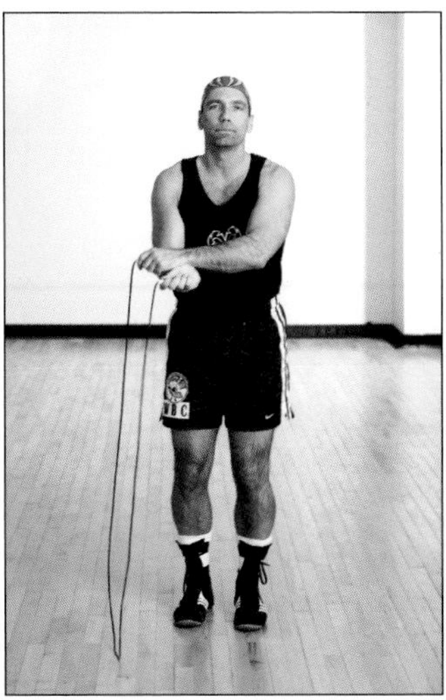

Figure 8–rope at one side

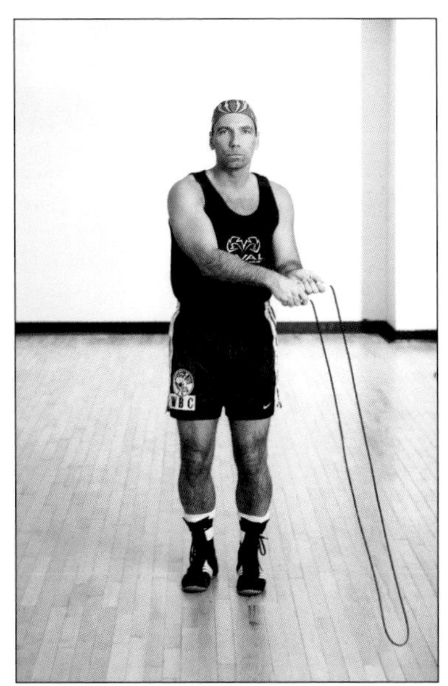

Figure 8–rope at the other side

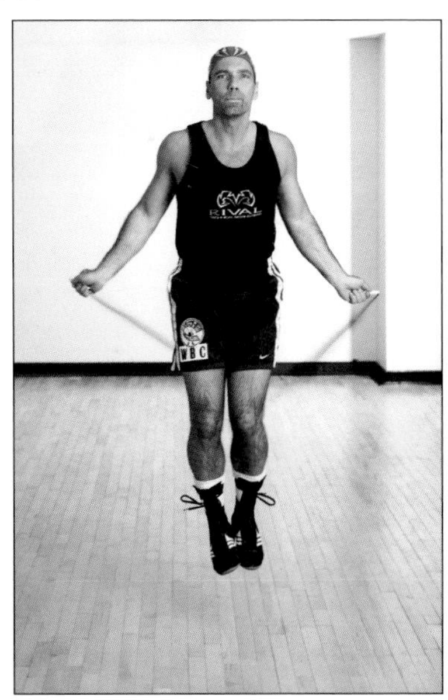

Figure 8–jump through

Move the rope from side to side, and then jump through the center. Working the rope in a neutral figure eight, move it from one side to the other in front of the body. Elbows are in close to the body, and the hands are close together. It is important to open the hands, so that the rope is in the proper position to jump through. Repeat the figure eight once, then jump through the rope. Repeat. One figure eight, one jump through the rope. The trick here is not to allow the hands to cross because this causes the rope to tangle and wrap around itself.

To start, try to perform basic jumps between 120 to 160 jumps per minute. The speed of the rope rotations and your height will influence the number of skips per minute performed. Work on the basics, and the more difficult and intricate jump roping will come easily.

Common Mistakes and Training Tips

Mistake: The feet keep get tangled in the rope.

Tip: The hands should be lower by your sides of the body with the elbows tucked in. Use only your wrists and forearms, not your shoulders, to turn the rope. Keep your eyes straight ahead. Looking at your feet can stress your neck muscles and changes the arc of the rope.

Mistake: Unable to learn new jumps.

Tip: Deconstruct the move down into the three-step breakdown. (1) Practice the jump without the rope. (2) Hold the rope in one hand only, rotating it off to one side, and practice the jump with the rope rotation. (3) Now jump through the rope practicing the new jump.

Mistake: Staying in one place.

Tip: Boxers are always moving. Once you have the basics down, move around.

The Boxer's Workout

7

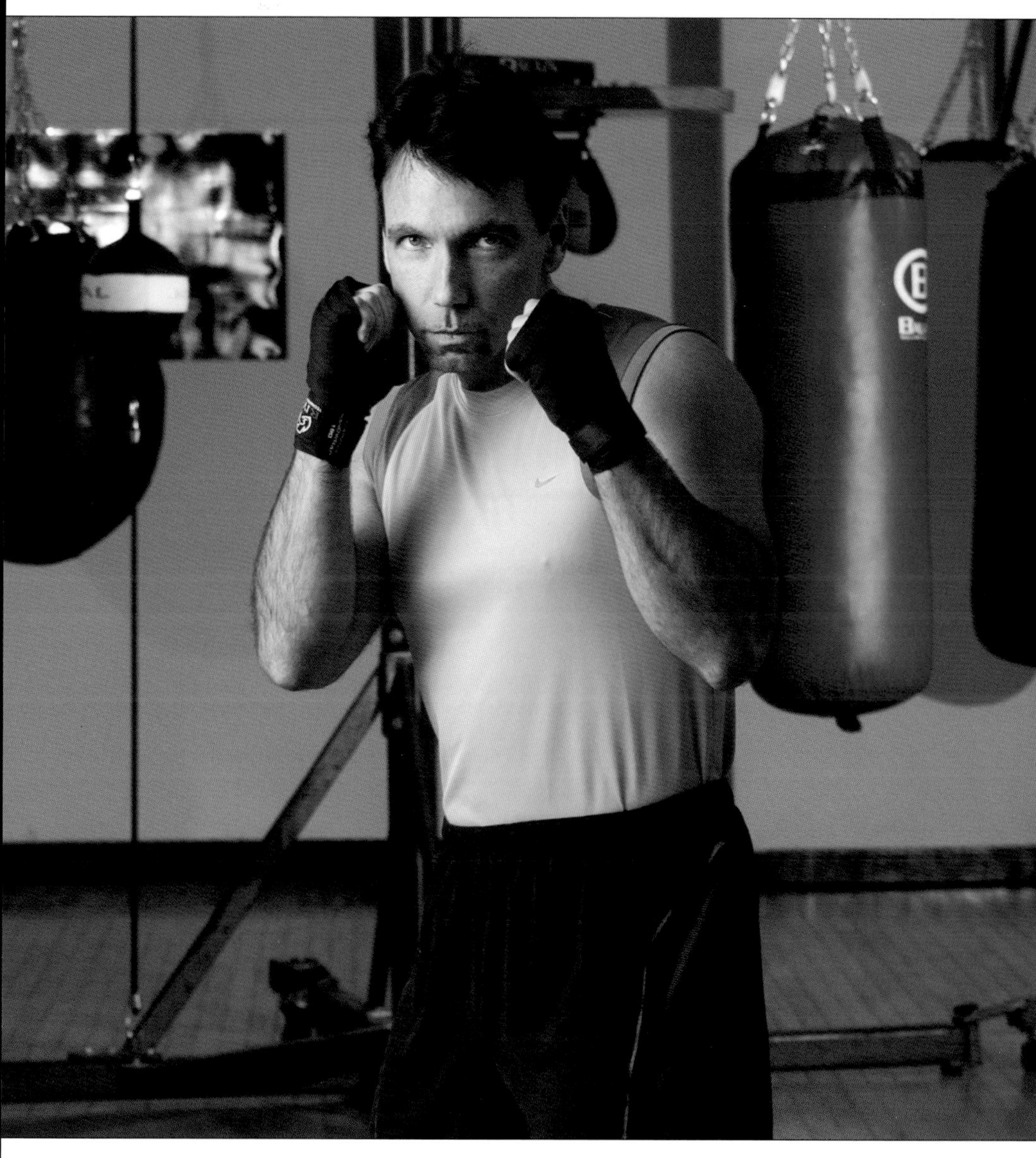

The Boxer's Workout is the basis of the Old School Boxing Workout and offers descriptions, guidelines, and skill level options to apply to your workout. Once you have mastered the Boxer's Workout, two other workouts are described. The "Champ's Workout," a definite challenge, is the next step up from the Boxer's Workout, and "Boxing Shorts," a thirty-minute maintenance program providing a quick, rigorous, and invigorating training session. Easy reference charts are presented at the end of the chapter.

The weight training and cardio workouts of the Old School Boxing Workout complement your training on boxing days. The power behind your punches on the heavy bag, the slipping and movement around the double-end bag, the muscle endurance needed for the speed bag, and the cardio-conditioning required to last the three-minute rounds are worked on during the weight and cardio training sessions.

The fluid agility of lightweight boxers and the heart stopping power of heavyweights can be yours without having to step into the ring. The Boxer's Workout pulls it all together: shadow boxing, bag work, skipping, target mitts, and core training. Grab your gloves and let's get into championship shape!

The Warm Up (Three minutes)

To get ready for the Boxer's Workout, become both mentally and physically prepared. As discussed in Chapter Three, shadow boxing is a great way to warm up the muscles, review the execution of the punches, and prepare yourself mentally to hit the different bags and target mitts. If a mirror is available, check out your stance, making sure the fists are held high, the elbows are in to protect the body, and you are in the classic boxing position. Keep the hands up and move around, side to side, front and back. Add some body movement and head movement. Now add some jabs and straight punches. Move around as if you were in the ring, not only throwing but evading punches as well. Stay loose and in control. Continue the shadow boxing warm-up for three minutes, and stretch after (refer to Chapter 8). Slowly take the limbs through a greater range of motion, and lengthen out the muscles. The major areas of concern are the shoulder area, hip flexor, and legs.

Shadow Boxing (two x three-minute rounds)

Now it's time to get more serious and execute the punches with a little more intent. As with the warm-up, move around, mix up the punches, and keep the heart rate elevated. Working in three-minute rounds, with one-minute rest in between, have a game plan of the punches and punch combinations you want to tackle. Develop both offensive moves and defensive moves. This is when you want to be creative and also work on transitions that do not feel comfortable and smooth. During shadow boxing, the punching technique, balance, weight transfers from foot to foot, and combinations can be developed and corrected. Get a feel for the three-minute time limit, and pace yourself so you are working at about 60 to 70 percent of your maximum effort. During the one-minute rest, take time to prepare for the next three-minute round. Ask yourself which punches felt smooth and under control, which movements did and did not flow well, and develop a strategy.

Follow these guidelines to match your shadow boxing rounds with your skill level:

Beginner

Perform the straight punches: the jab and the straight right power punch. Concentrate on the punch execution and placement of the arms, the wrist, and the body. Add some footwork and punch combinations, and focus mainly on the technique of the punches until they become second nature.

Intermediate

Perform a greater variety of punches and punch combinations, adding footwork and body movement. Also, increase the intensity by adding a bounce to the movement and snap to your punches.

Advanced

Take the workout up a notch, moving faster with more combinations and fancier footwork. Snap the punches and keep the pace fast for the entire three minutes. You can also perform the same movement as the intermediate level and hold onto small weights (two to three pounds). If holding hand weights for punching, punch at 60 percent intensity, developing muscular and punching endurance. Use your imagination, and work on both attacking and retreating moves.

Jump Rope (twelve minutes)

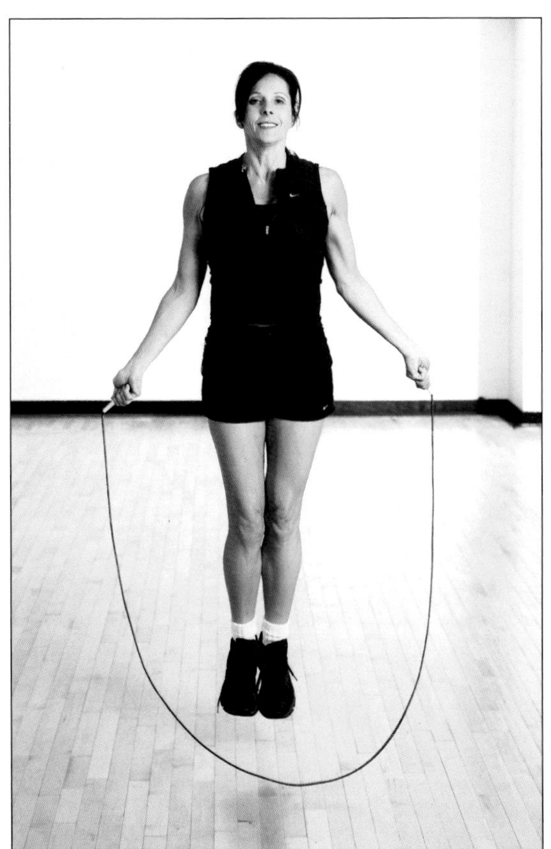

Start jumping rope at an easy pace. The footwork should be kept basic and the intensity low for about two minutes. Increase the intensity slightly by either performing more intricate footwork or by increasing the speed at which you are jumping. If you are beginning, divide the jumping rope into four three-minute rounds and build up to one twelve–minute continuous round. If you are a seasoned jumper, you may want to try some sprints (around the six-minute mark), perform high knee jogging, twenty to twenty-five seconds and then bring the intensity back down for sixty to ninety seconds. Repeat four to six times. Attempt to jump for a total of twelve minutes. This can be accomplished by working up to the time frame, taking a break when needed, or by reducing the intensity until you have build up your stamina. Remember when trying new moves to use the three-step breakdown (Refer to Chapter 6).

Heavy Bag (three x three-minute rounds)

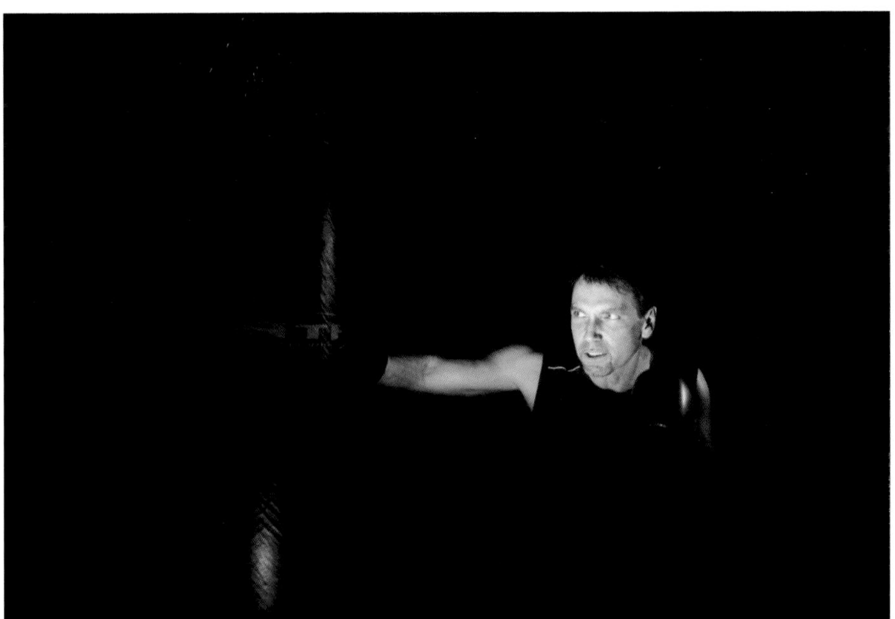

Three different intensity levels are described from beginner to more advanced. Choose one that is best suited to your fitness level and experience.

Level One: Just Starting Out

If you have never hit a heavy bag before, this is a great place to learn the technique and power of landing a punch. By performing repetition after repetition of a single punch, the movement and execution will become second nature. This will set you up for adding movement and combinations so they flow easily. Start punching for a total of two minutes, working up to three minutes for all three rounds. Rest between each round for one minute, walking around the bag and reducing the heart rate slightly. Regroup and plan you next attack.

Round One

This round is a "range finder" and allows you to get the feel of hitting the bag and the power behind the punches. Standing in the classic boxing stance, keep you hands up, practice throwing your left jab and moving to the left or right.

Round Two

Standing in the classic boxing stance, practice your straight right power punch. After you obtain the range with the straight right, put it together with the jab, for a one-two, (left-jab/straight-right combination). Add movement to the right or left, after the punch combinations.

Round Three

Start setting the punch tempo with your jab. Throw five to six sharp jabs moving and circling the bag in both directions. Now throw a one-two, move around and repeat. Find your rhythm. (Jab-move-jab-move-jab-move-jab-move-jab-one-two).

Level Two: Intermediate

In this level, you should feel comfortable working on the bag performing the basic punches. Put together combinations, adding body movement and footwork. This will increase the intensity of the workout. If you are comfortable with two-minute rounds, then it is time to bump it up to three minutes. Rest for one minute keep moving and walk around during the rest period. Focus on the next round.

Round One

Punch the bag with the sharp left jabs and one-two combinations. Move around, work on balance, and incorporate footwork.

Round Two

Punch with more intent. Add slips, feints, and stay light on your feet. Add some body punches, jabs and one-two's. Use your legs to lower and raise your punches. For example, try some double jabs, move away from the bag, move towards the bag, and finish with a one-two punch.

Round Three

Add some hooks to the mix. For example: One-two-hook Combination. Step into the bag as you launch your left jab followed by a straight right. You should now be in a position to throw a short left hook to finish the combination. Step away and circle the bag as you plan your next sequence of punches.

Become aware of your timing and find your own rhythm. Maintain a center of balance when you make contact on the bag with a maximum hit.

Level Three: Advanced

Once you have the punches down, work on the bag as if you were in the ring. Add more movement, have a strategy (game plan), and work in hooks, uppercuts with jabs, and power punches. Mix it all up. Hit the bag for three-minute rounds and rest for one minute.

For the most intense three-round sessions follow these guidelines:

Round One

Throw plenty of jabs to start the round off. Use your legs to get in and out of range: "Punch and get out." Put together two- and three-punch combinations developing smooth transitions from one punch to the next. Work at 60 to 70 percent of full intent.

Round Two

Add more power and intent to the punches. Work in flurries, six, seven, or eight rapid-fire punches. Keep moving around after your flurries: jab and move, jab and move. Try to add flurries three to four times per round.

Round Three

Put it all together. Remember, nothing stays still in the boxing ring, so keep moving, change direction, and use the heavy bag to your advantage. Work your "punches in bunches."

Heavy-Bag Speed Sprints

This advanced punching workout on the heavy bag trains for punch speed, works the arm and back muscles for power and endurance, and challenges the cardiovascular system. Start with fifteen-second sprints, working up to 20-second sprints. It is best to have a timer. Always rest the same amount of time as you work. Walk around and think about your next sprint. Repeat three to four more times. (For more sprint options refer to Chapter 4.)

Beginner:

Sprint 1:	15 seconds	Rest:	15 seconds
Sprint 2:	15 seconds	Rest:	15 seconds
Sprint 3:	15 seconds	Rest:	15 seconds

Target Mitts (three x three-minute rounds)

If you have a partner, train with target mitts. Concentrate on the execution of the punches, work for three three-minute rounds, alternating catching and throwing with your partner. Focus on speed, technique and proper execution. (Refer to Chapter 5).

Beginner:

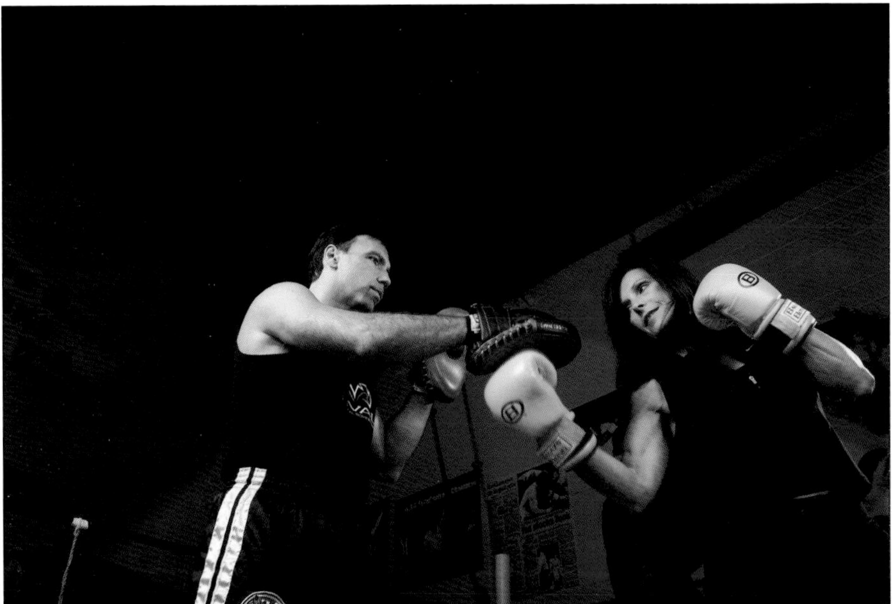

Puncher

Practice left jabs, finding your range. Focus on the punch execution and placement of the arms, the wrist, and the body. Add straight right power punches, listening for the catchers commands and keeping your eye on the target. The left jab goes to the left target mitt of the catcher, and the straight right goes to the right target mitt of the catcher. Punch and get out, using the legs to move forward and back, side to side.

Catcher

The catcher calls out the punch commands, holding the target mitts one and a half feet to two feet away from the body, arms slightly bent at the elbow in a semi-tense position. In the classic boxing stance, keep the puncher in view, the elbows bent slightly, and meet the punch.

Intermediate:

Puncher

Perform a greater variety of punches and punch combinations, including hooks and uppercuts. React quickly to the punch commands being called by the catcher.

Catcher

Become comfortable with catching a variety of punches and punch combinations. Set the tempo, moving the puncher around and ensuring the mitt is ready for the next punch in the combination.

Advanced:

Puncher

Work on four- and five-punch combinations, include slipping in the combinations. Good balance and good footwork will be the keys to success.

Catcher

Develop and call commands working on both attacking and retreating moves. Communicate well with the puncher.

Ladder Drills on the Heavy Bag (optional)

If you do not have access to target mitts or a partner, perform ladders drills on the heavy bag with the left jab, straight right and one-two's. Refer to Chapter 4.

Cardio Cool-Down Round

The purpose of the cool-down is to decrease the heart rate and to review the punches. If you have a speed-bag and double-end bag available, this is a great time to work out on them. Refer to Chapter 4 for information on speed-bag and double-end bag training. End with shadow boxing for three to six minutes, punching with light intent, rather than focusing on power. Stay light on your feet, shrugging and rotating the shoulders. Let the muscles relax.

Abdominal Workout

Now that you have cooled down and your heart rate has decreased, perform abdominal exercises as described in Chapter 9. Concentrate on a controlled execution of the exercises, contracting the abdominal muscles and focusing on the body core muscles.

Cooldown/Stretches

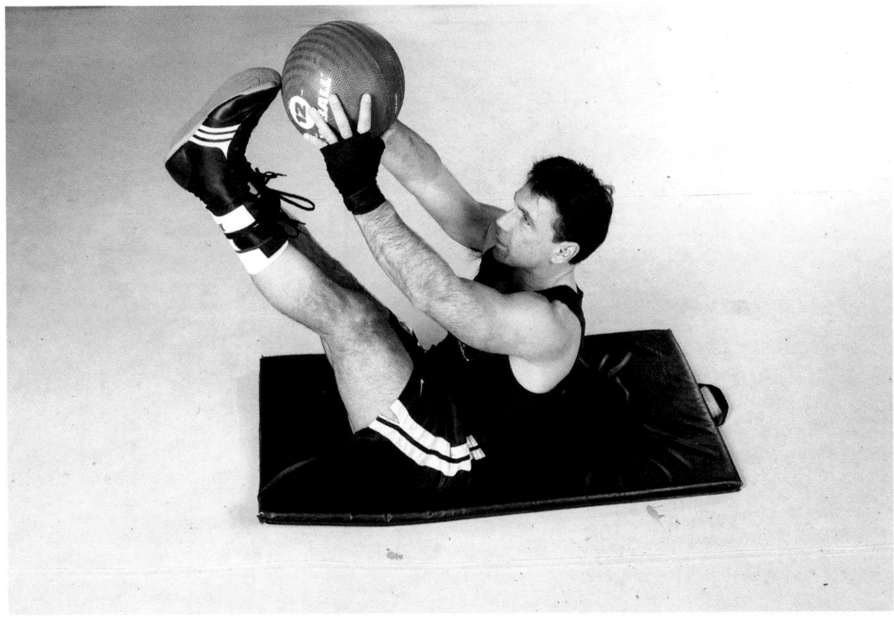

The stretches are described in Chapter 8. After every workout, perform stretching and flexibility exercises. This will help lengthen the muscle fibers and reduce soreness the next day.

The Boxer's Workout

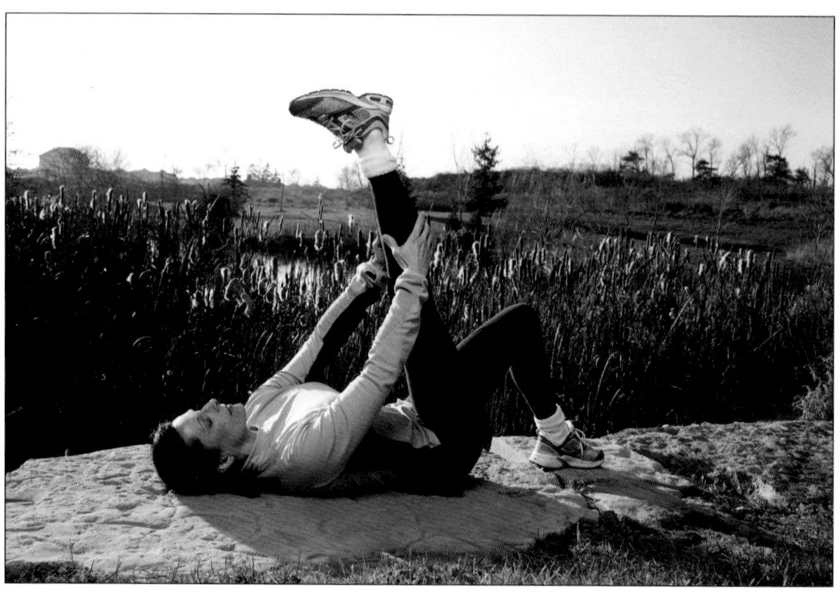

Warm-up Round (three minutes)

Shadow box practicing the basic punches focusing on technique and execution. Perform light stretching after.

Shadow Boxing (two x three-minute rounds)

Choose the beginner, intermediate, or advanced level and work at two three-minute rounds.

Round One: Add more movement while throwing the punches and combinations.

Round Two: Add more intent to the punches, and work on combinations.

Jump Rope (twelve minutes)

Jump at a moderate pace for two to three minutes, gradually increasing the difficulty, mixing up the tempo and footwork, for a total of twelve minutes (refer to Chapter 6).

Heavy Bag (three x three-minute rounds)

Choose the appropriate level to work at according to your fitness level and experience.

Work the punches on the heavy bag for three minutes and rest for one minute in between. Perform three rounds.

Heavy Bag Speed Sprints

Face the heavy bag straight on, check your arm reach, relax the legs, keep the body core tight, and start punching. Remember to rest the same length of time as the sprint.

Sprint 1: 15 to 20 seconds (rest 15 to 20 seconds)
Sprint 2: 15 to 20 seconds (rest 15 to 20 seconds)
Sprint 3: 15 to 20 seconds (rest 15 to 20 seconds)

Target Mitts (three x three-minute rounds)

Partner work, alternating rounds, catching and punching. Choose the beginner, intermediate, or advanced level, according to your fitness level and experience. Concentrate on the punches, working for three three-minute rounds each.

Ladder Drills on the Heavy Bag (optional)

If you do not have access to target mitts or a partner, perform ladders drills with the left, straight right and one-twos. Refer to the Chapter 4.

Cool-down Round (three to six minutes)

Shadow box lightly, moving around, and review the punches. Practice on the double-end bag and speed bag if available.

Abdominal Workout (six minutes)

Refer to Chapter 9, Muscle Conditioning. Sample sequence: Thirty abdominal crunches, thirty oblique crunches...repeat three times. Two sets of twenty-five abdominal leg presses. Body plank: forty-five seconds to ninety seconds.

Cool-down/Stretches (five to seven minutes)

Refer to Chapter 8, "Cardio-Conditioning." Spend five to ten minutes performing these exercises.

The Champ's Workout

If you have successfully been training at the boxer's workout level, then give the Champ's Workout a try!

Warm-up Round (three minutes)

Shadow box practicing the basic punches focusing on technique and execution. Perform light stretches after.

Shadow Boxing (three x three-minute rounds)

Optional: Use hand weights two to three pounds.
Round One: Practice the basic punches focusing on technique and execution.
Round Two: Put combinations together, adding head movement and developing fluidity between the punches and combinations.
Round Three: No weights. Work all the punches together adding lots of footwork.

Jump Rope (twelve to twenty minutes)

Warm-up: Easy jumping for two minutes
Skip: Normal rate for two to four minutes
Sprint: Twenty double skips
Skip: Normal rate for two to four minutes
Sprint: Thirty double skips
Skip: Normal rate for two to four minutes
Sprint: Forty double skips
Skip: Easy skipping two to four minutes
Note: If you have not mastered double jumps, perform high knees at a faster pace.

Heavy Bag (four x three-minute rounds)

Work for three minutes and rest for one minute.

Round One: Mix up the punches, add footwork, and work on combinations.

Round Two: Burnout drill: five second speed sprint move around for fifteen seconds, repeat for the three-minute round.

Round Three: Work the bag as if you were in the ring. Punches in bunches.

Round Four: Punch for power for five seconds, move around the bag for fifteen seconds, and repeat the sprint again for a total of three minutes.

THE CHAMP'S WORKOUT

OPTION ONE **PARTNER WORK**	OPTION TWO **NO PARTNER OPTION**
TARGET MITTS (3 x3 minute rounds) Alternate rounds catching and punching.	**LADDERS** Perform drills with left jab, straight right and one-two's. Refer to Chapter 4
TARGET MITT SPEED DRILLS	**HEAVY BAG SPEED SPRINTS**
Straight punches – 20 seconds	Face the heavy bag straight on, check your arm reach, relax the legs. Sprint and rest the same amount of time.
Hooks – 20 seconds Uppercuts – 20 seconds Repeat twice before switching partners. (One drill per person)	Sprint 1: 40 seconds (rest 40 seconds) Sprint 2: 40 seconds (rest 40 seconds) Sprint 3: 30 seconds (rest 30 seconds) Sprint 4: 30 seconds (rest 30 seconds) Sprint 5: 20 seconds (rest 20 seconds) Sprint 6: 20 seconds (rest 20 seconds)

Speed Bag (six minutes)

Final blast on your shoulders.

Double-end Bag (two x three-minute rounds)

Include rapid-succession punching, combinations, and defensive moves. Refer to Chapter 4.

Cool-down Round (one x three-minute round)

Shadow box for three minutes, moving around and throwing lightly.

Abdominal Workout

Refer to Chapter 9, Muscle Conditioning.

Sample sequence:

Abdominal crunches: Thirty reps

Medicine ball basic curl ups: Thirty reps

Supine cycle: Thirty reps

Medicine ball oblique twists: Thirty reps

Hip raises without medicine ball: Thirty reps.

Cool-down/Stretches (five to seven minutes)

Refer to Chapter 8. Always stretch after each workout.

"Boxing Shorts": A 30 Minute Maintenance Workout

There are times when you may not have time for a full workout, or after completing the twelve-week program you may feel like a change. Try the thirty-minute maintenance work-out "Boxing Shorts". It allows you to maintain your existing fitness level in a shorter workout and gives you the opportunity to throw plenty of punches. The Boxing Shorts workout should not replace the Boxer's Workout on a continual basis, but it is great for a change. It is rigorous and invigorating, and it challenges the cardiovascular and muscular systems.

Keep moving from exercise to exercise, staying focused and not taking any breaks. The program design is short enough for anyone with a busy schedule.

Warm-up Round (three minutes)

Start with an easy warm-up shadow boxing with light hand weights, not heavier than two pounds. If you have a speed bag, work for two to three minutes on it. Take the muscles and the joints through an optimal range of motion. Wrap your hands.

Jump Rope (eight minutes)

Jump rope, keeping a good jumping rate and lifting the knees high. Try some varied footwork. Keep the pace of jumping fairly fast. Perform some sprints and double jumps to elevate the heart rate.

Heavy Bag (two x five-minute rounds) (one minute rest in between and at the end of the round)

The body has most likely adapted to the three-minute rounds. By increasing the length of time boxing, you place an overload on the muscles and energy sources. To really increase the workout, try to hit the bag at a three-minute pace for five minutes.

Muscle Conditioning (three minutes)

Squats: Overhead or power squats with a medicine ball. Three sets of twenty to twenty-five reps. Add forward lunges if there is time. Refer to Chapter 9.

Abdominal Workout (four minutes)

Perform abdominal exercises with the medicine ball. Sample sequence: 40 curl-ups, twenty pullover sit-ups, forty hip crunches. Repeat two times. Refer to Chapter 9.

Cool down/Stretches (two Minutes)

Perform stretches and flexibility exercises as described in Chapter 8.

Cardio Conditioning and Stretching 8

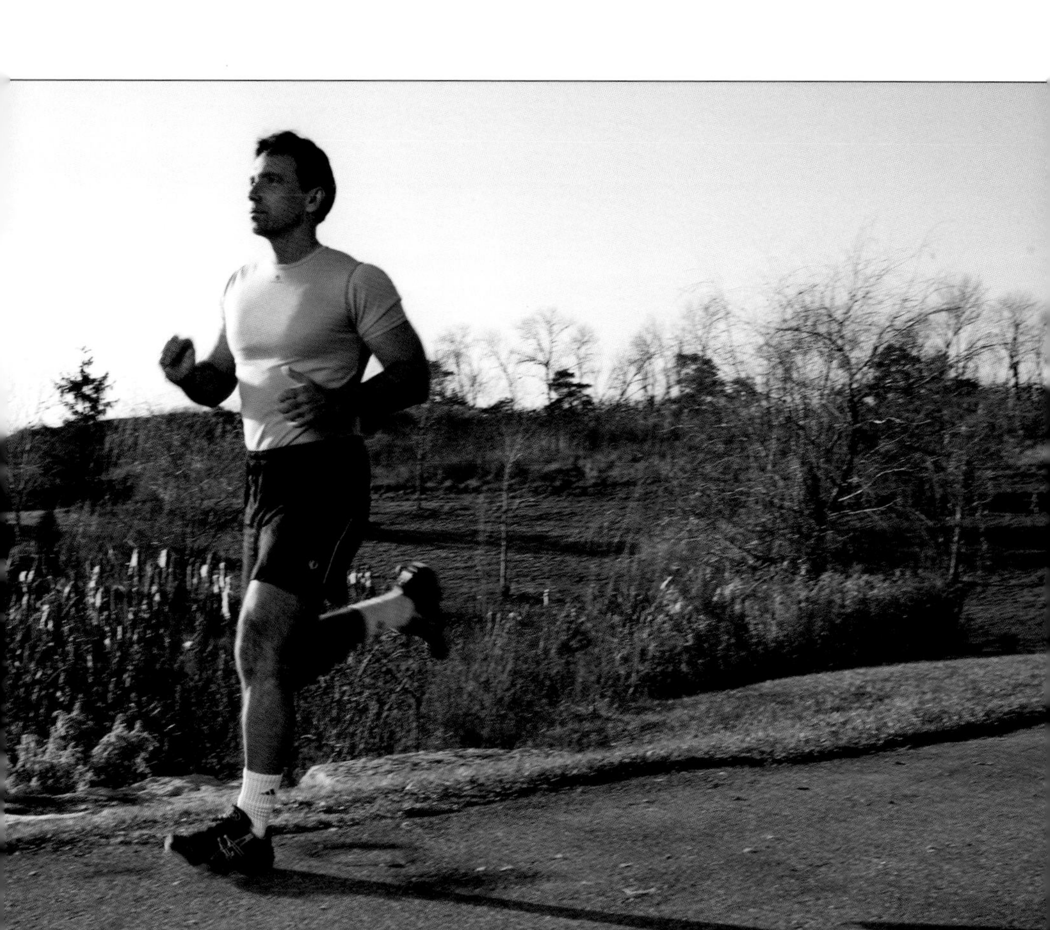

Cardio Conditioning

People were designed to move, to place one foot in front of the other, to develop their muscles, and to expand their physical and mental capabilities. Running can be done just about everywhere and with very little equipment or experience. Just a pair of shoes and the desire to move your body from one place to another is all that is needed. Running can be done in a group and be a very social activity, or it can be performed on an individual basis. The training is specific to each individual, and you will find your preferred routes, time of day, speed, and tempo.

Cardio conditioning days in the Old School Boxing Workout improve the ability of the heart and lungs to adapt to the external demands placed on the body during physical activity. If you prefer not to, or are unable to run outdoors, then substitute the time on cardio equipment such as a treadmill, an elliptical machine, or a stationary bike. You could also jump rope at a moderate pace. If you are coming off a mild injury, you may replace the cardio conditioning days with an activity that will increase your heart rate and breathing rate for the recommended length of time, such as swimming.

Why and How a Boxer Does It

Both the respiratory and cardiovascular systems must be trained in order to "go the distance" in a boxing round. Depending on whether the fight is an amateur or a professional fight, and no one is knocked out in the first few rounds, the boxer has to keep moving from twelve minutes to forty minutes.

To build the necessary stamina, boxers usually train their cardio systems by running, jumping rope, and hitting the bag. The roadwork portion of their training involves running at a relatively moderate pace, usually outdoors. Roadwork training generally is performed three to four times per week, with the intention of building stamina to stay strong through the entire bout.

Start with roadwork (or the equivalent on a bike, treadmill, or elliptical machine) to condition the aerobic capacity of the body. As you become more adapted to the distance and pace of the roadwork, the cardiovascular and respiratory systems will improve. More demands can then be placed on the body during the training in order to develop an even higher level of fitness.

Traditionally, cardio training for boxers included long runs and also the interval training from sparring with a partner in the ring. The long runs trained the cardio-aerobic system, the system that utilizes oxygen as the source of energy and allows an activity to be continued for an extended period of time. Working in the ring and sparring with a partner accomplished the training for the cardio-anaerobic system. The anaerobic system requires glucose, adenosine tri-phosphate (ATP) and creatine phosphate (CP) as the energy sources to perform the activity and provide quick strong movements for shorter periods of time. This type of activity can only be performed in short spurts and is known as interval training.

Long runs, skipping, and sparring with a partner in the ring were the accepted methods to train the cardiovascular and respiratory systems—that is until recently! Many are realizing the importance of imitating the demands of the three-minute round by performing running sprints and interval training outside of the ring. Remember, a three-minute round places specific demands on the body, which needs to be trained to respond to the faster and more intense demands of each single round, as well as to the endurance requirements to last the entire fight.

Measuring Training Intensities

To start a running program, it is necessary to learn how to measure the level at which you are working. There are a few methods that are standard to the fitness industry and easily applied to cardio conditioning. The heart rate and "talk test" are two ways to measure how hard you are working.

The Heart Rate

The heart beats a specific number of times per minute, and this number is unique to each individual. When the body starts to move during an activity, the heart muscle must pump more blood more often to provide sufficient quantities of oxygen to the muscle tissue. A trained heart pumps out a greater volume of blood and does not need to beat as often to provide the necessary oxygen to the body whether at rest or while exercising. Many factors such as age, heredity, and sex cannot be changed, but your fitness level can. As your cardio conditioning improves, your heart rate will decrease, so that there are fewer beats per minute.

How to Take Your Pulse

To take your resting heart rate without equipment, sit in a comfortable position and find either your carotid artery (in the neck region) or your radial artery (on the inside of the wrist). The pulse in the neck area is found by gently placing the index finger and/or the middle finger at the side of the neck, just beside the trachea. It is important not to press too hard because arteries are pressure sensitive, and the heart rate may actually drop. The radial pulse in the wrist can be found by placing the index and middle fingers on the underside of the wrist and the thumb on the top of the wrist. Once again, press lightly.

To measure your heart rate when exercising, reduce your intensity and find your pulse. Press lightly and count for a specific length of time, somewhere between ten and sixty seconds. If you count for ten seconds, then multiply the number by six, if you take a thirty-second count, then multiply by two. The longer sixty-second count is the most precise. Nevertheless, to count for sixty seconds means that you will have to reduce your activity during the time, disrupting your workout.

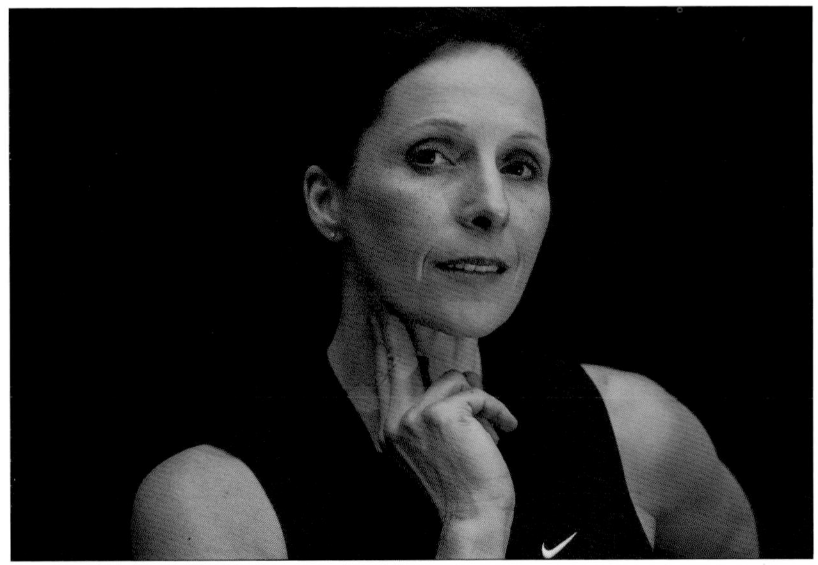

Carotid pulse

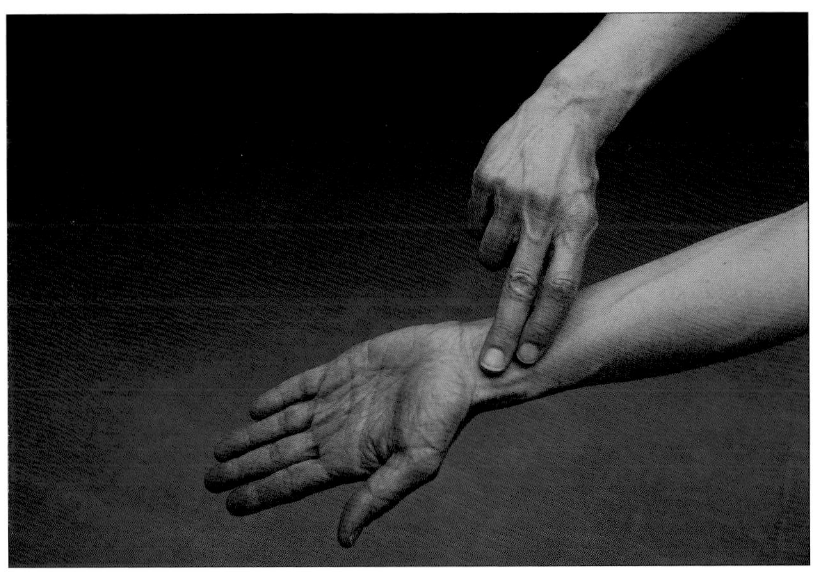

Radial pulse

Heart Rate Monitors

Today's digital heart rate monitors, usually incorporated into a training watch or stopwatch, are available at most sporting goods stores. A special electrode sensor is placed on the arm or the chest and picks up the signal of the heart beating. These are great devices because you do not have to stop exercising to take a pulse. And they are generally accurate. Excessive motion when the electrode makes contact with the skin surface, however, may produce inaccurate readings. Also, other electromagnetic systems may interfere with the heart signal.

The Resting Heart Rate

The resting heart rate is a good indicator of your basic fitness level and is a great starting place to learn about your current fitness level. Just before you get out of bed in the morning, count the number of times that your heart beats in one minute. This number is known as your resting heart rate and is the base measurement indicator to determine improvements in your fitness level. As your fitness level improves, the resting heart rate will decrease, meaning that the heart does not have to pump as many times per minute to provide the body with oxygen-rich blood.

The Training Heart Rate

The training heart rate is a number range in which the heart should be beating in order to produce a conditioning effect. To obtain a training effect on the heart muscle, a general rule of thumb is to maintain a heart rate that is between 60 and 75 percent of your maximum heart rate. One method of calculating the maximum heart rate is by subtracting your age from 220. Therefore, if you are thirty years old, your maximum heart rate will be 220 minus thirty or 190 beats in sixty seconds. Sixty percent of the maximum heart will rate will give the lower heart rate number for the training heart rate. In our example, 60 percent of 190 beats equals 114 beats per minute. Seventy-five percent of the maximum heart rate will give you the higher end of the training heart rate, or 75 percent of 190 beats equals 142 beats in a minute. The training heart rate would therefore be 114 beats to 142 beats per minute.

The intensity level at which you train should be specific to you individually and is dependent on both your own individual capabilities and the type of exercise being performed. Ensure that the level you at which work exceeds mild physical demand, but does not produce extreme breathlessness, fatigue, or confusion.

During cardio conditioning, as the heart is trained, its rate readings over a period of training weeks should decrease. Let's say that during week one, after twenty minutes of roadwork, the heart rate count for sixty seconds was 140 beats per minute. In week four, performing exactly the same route and time duration the heart rate may be reduced to 138 to 135 beats per minute. Generally, a decrease of four to ten beats per minute can be expected after a six-to-eight week training period. A less fit individual will see a greater difference, whereas a well-conditioned athlete will see less of a difference. Some variables such as age, initial fitness level, length of training program, and program intensity will influence the training results.

The method you select to determine your heart rate should be consistent from workout to workout, so that comparisons are valid. Many factors may influence your heart rate from day to day such as stress level, digestion, biological rhythms, temperature, and your health status. The heart-rate measure should only be a guide when assessing the differences in your cardio-fitness level over a period of time.

The "Talk Test" Measure of Exercise Intensity

An easy way to measure how hard you are working is to use the "talk test." This is a very subjective measure of the workout intensity and can be very useful in determining the comfort zone of aerobic intensity. To determine your talking threshold, increase your activity until it is difficult to talk and breathe comfortably. This is the talking threshold. You want to be just below this level. The aim is to breathe rhythmically and comfortably throughout all phases of the workout. As you progress to higher functional capacities and higher workout levels, the talk test is a conservative measure, especially at more than 80 percent of the functional capacity. It is more accurate to use a heart rate monitor.

Equipment

Footwear

The most important purchase you will make is a functional and comfortable pair of running shoes. The shoe protects and supports the foot and improves traction when running. There are a variety of styles and brand names to choose from today, and you're sure to find a fit that is specific to your lifestyle and running style. Running is a straight-ahead heel strike activity that produces a force many times that of your body weight. The shoe should have sufficient support for your weight and provide adequate sole cushioning. Good heel support and mid sole flexibility are two important factors to look for in a running shoe. Visit a store that has knowledgable and trained staff, try on different styles, and make an educated purchase.

Clothing

As a rule of thumb, in hot weather wear light-colored cotton or breathable fabrics, which are loose fitting. In cold weather, try to dress in layers, and cover the head, face, and hands. A great investment to make is in clothing that has moisture-transport capabilities. The high-tech fibers in the clothes allow perspiration (water vapor) to evaporate away from the skin and out through the material, but they do not allow rain droplets to soak into the material. Some of the fabrics combine water repellency, wind-proofing, and warming properties for colder outside training.

Standard Precautions

Meals

Try not to train the cardio system for at least nienty minutes after a full meal. A large meal will require the heart to pump blood and oxygen to the stomach and the intestines to assist in the digestion of food. When you start to exercise, the heart must pump blood to the working muscles, leaving less oxygen available for the brain and the digestion of food. The result can be nausea, gastric discomfort, increased stress on the heart muscle and an ineffective workout. The length of time between a meal and a cardio workout is specific to the amount of food eaten and the intensity of the workout. The larger the meal, the longer you should wait before you run.

Illness

Strenuous cardio exercising should be avoided with flu or upper respiratory tract infections. If you are on prescription medications or over-the-counter medicine, consult with your doctor as to whether there are any contraindications of the medicine when combined with moderate and/or intense physical activity.

Pollution

Be aware of the pollution index and consider training indoors, especially if you have any upper respiratory weaknesses.

Hot Weather

Reduce your exercise intensity if you are training in very hot or humid weather conditions or at altitudes higher than 5000 feet above sea level. Wear comfortable, loose-fitting clothing with moisture transport capabilities. You may need a hat for cooling and UV protection. You'll want to protect your eyes from UV rays as well. Select sunglasses that won't slip down your nose when you start to sweat. Protecting your eyes and face from the sun will help keep you relaxed, so that you can focus on your run. Avoid training during the hottest part of the day and stay out of direct sunlight if possible. Drink water before, during, and after exercising. Avoid alcohol and caffeinated beverages (alcohol, tea, and colas act as diuretics and can actually increase fluid loss). Stay in your training heart rate zone because your working heart rate may increase faster due to the heat. Reduce your exercising intensity. You may not be running as far or as fast as usual, but you are working just as hard.

How to Stay Cool:

- It usually takes a week or two to adjust to any major jump in temperature.
- Be well hydrated before your workout. Eight to twelve cups of water a day is normal for an active person.
- Avoid exercising during the hottest part of the day. Do so in the morning or evening when it's milder.
- Pace yourself. Replace lost body fluids by drinking four to six ounces in twenty-minute intervals during your run.

Cold Weather

Plenty of discipline is needed to run in cold weather because there are many reasons not to go out for a run. Focus on the end result and meet the challenge. Avoid training outside on extremely windy and icy days or in temperatures below–10 degrees Celsius or 15 degrees Fahrenheit.

Layer your clothes. Wear fabrics with moisture transport qualities next to your skin and a breathable windproof suit on the outside. Another layer should be added on very cold days. Up to 50 percent of the body's heat is lost through the head, so wear a balaclava or toque to keep warm. Wear mitts or gloves on your hands. If you find breathing cold air uncomfortable, wear a covering over your month and nose to warm up the air. Wear sunscreen and sunglasses to protect the face and the eyes from the glare of the snow-covered ground.

Warm up thoroughly and start at a comfortable pace. Shorten your stride to improve your footing on icy roads. It doesn't matter whether or not you cover the same distance you might on a summer's day. Keep your speed work for dry, indoor surfaces.

Decide on a time rather than distance. If you are running in a desolate area, run with a group. If you are by yourself, find a route that you can cut short and where help is readily available.

It is important to remember that a great performance is only possible with every element being met. On some days, however, not all the elements are in our control. The best you can do is to prepare yourself both physically and mentally and work to your personal potential. Many of our best runs have occurred at temperatures well below freezing and on snow-covered trails.

Trail Running

Sometimes it's great to just to go for a run, not timing yourself, or measuring distances. And, if you get the opportunity to run on trails, away from the city streets, another world is opened up. Take the opportunity to look around and take in some of the beauty of nature. Time passes without much effort, the muscles are challenged differently, and the stresses of the week dissipate quickly. This type of running experience can be exhilarating and very rewarding.

The Cardio Program

Part of the cardio-conditioning program includes training for endurance—to go the distance—and the long run will be an essential part of this program. It is important to note that these long runs serve as the foundation for overall conditioning and must be accomplished before moving onto the interval sprint work. During the continuous training, the objective is to sustain an aerobic activity for twenty to sixty minutes. Train at a moderate intensity level for both safety and comfort reasons. When the body's stamina is improved, fatigue will occur less often, and the chance of injury will be reduced. The physical condition of the body will then develop to a base level of fitness allowing greater physical demands to be placed on it. Once this base level of conditioning is achieved, then interval training can be incorporated into the cardio-conditioning program.

The cardio-conditioning days are day two and day four, and the workout session should last from thirty minutes to one hour. Depending on your base fitness level, the program may be started with a walk or jog, increasing up to a full jog, run, and sprint.

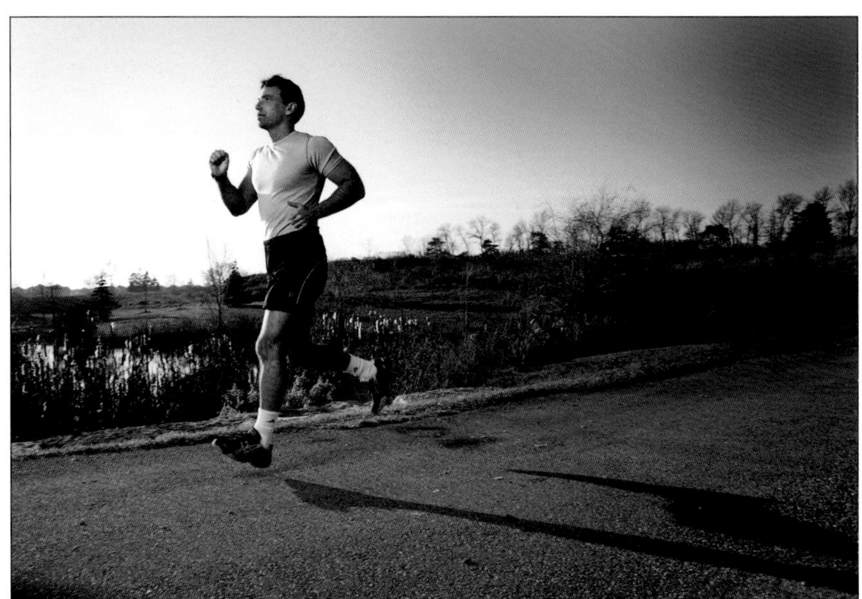

Effective Running Technique:

- The head stays upright with the chin in a neutral position.
- The shoulders are relaxed, down, and back.
- The arms swing straight forward and back. Keep your elbows bent at ninety degrees, and hold the hands partially open or in a relaxed fist. Minimize the arms crossing the body.

- The hips tip upwards, with the torso or core muscles held tight, giving support to the lower back.
- The knee moves horizontally. Avoid excessive up-and-down movement.
- For proper foot plant, let your foot fall directly below your knee, and then swing it forward.
- Minimize the contact time your foot has with ground. Strive for a quick turnover.
- Maintain a relaxed running position.

Cardio Conditioning Workout: Day Two & Day Four

The Warm-up

It is important to warm up before starting any running program. A great way to increase the blood flow in the body is to warm up by shadow boxing: Moving side to side and forwards and backwards, throwing punches. You can also warm up by walking for five minutes at a fairly good pace, swinging the arms and stretching out the muscles if they feel tight. Perform pre-activity stretches.

Initial Conditioning Level: Just Starting Out

The Run/Walk Method

Whether you are just starting out or you have been away from running for a while, the run-walk training method helps to build stamina, so that you can increase your total running time. This method of training reduces the chances of overuse injuries of the muscles and the joints. Before you know it, you'll be running longer and farther.

Begin by walking (two to five minutes) and jogging (two to five minutes), intermittently for a total of twelve to fifteen minutes. Try to work at 60 to 75 percent of your maximum heart rate or use the talk test, remembering that you should be able to talk while still breathing heavily. The walk breaks need to be done at a brisk rate in order to maintain an elevated heart rate. Your goal is to increase the total length of time of the walk and jog to thirty to forty-five minutes. Initially walk and jog in equal intervals, and then gradually increase the jogging interval to be longer than the walking interval. This initial conditioning stage may last between four to six weeks, sometimes longer.

Intermediate Conditioning Level: Improvement Stage

If you are currently involved in an exercise program or are comfortable running for twenty minutes continuously, then you are at a level at which you will be able to improve your running speed and distance over the next eight to twelve weeks. By gradually increasing the jogging distance and the speed, you are training the heart to be able to handle greater physical stresses. The heart should be working at 60 to 85 percent of the maximum rate. The time that you spend running can be increased every two to three weeks. Gradually increase the distance and time, and work up to continuous running/jogging for forty-five minutes to one hour.

Once you are comfortable with continuous training, then you can add interval training to your cardio-conditioning days. But you have to understand: You need to work up to it. Start to include sprints slowly and at a lower than maximum effort. Try including a few sprints in the fifth cardio-conditioning workout and every fourth workout after that. Refer to interval and sprint training under Advanced Conditioning Level.

Advanced Conditioning Level: Run Further...Run Faster!

This is the stage at which you are comfortable working in both continuous and interval training, and it is usually reached after the first six months of working out. As you jog farther and your cardiovascular or respiratory endurance improves, increase your stride frequency or the rate at which you place each foot on the ground. Run faster. Run farther. The workout should last for thirty to sixty minutes, working at a level of 75 to 85 percent of your maximum heart rate. For longer runs, stay focused and motivated. Running with a partner often helps. Keep your heart rate within your target training zone, applying the "talk test" method. If you can talk to someone without gasping, then you are working in your target zone. Add variety to your workout, performing intervals, track sprints, timed sprints, and hill training.

Interval Training

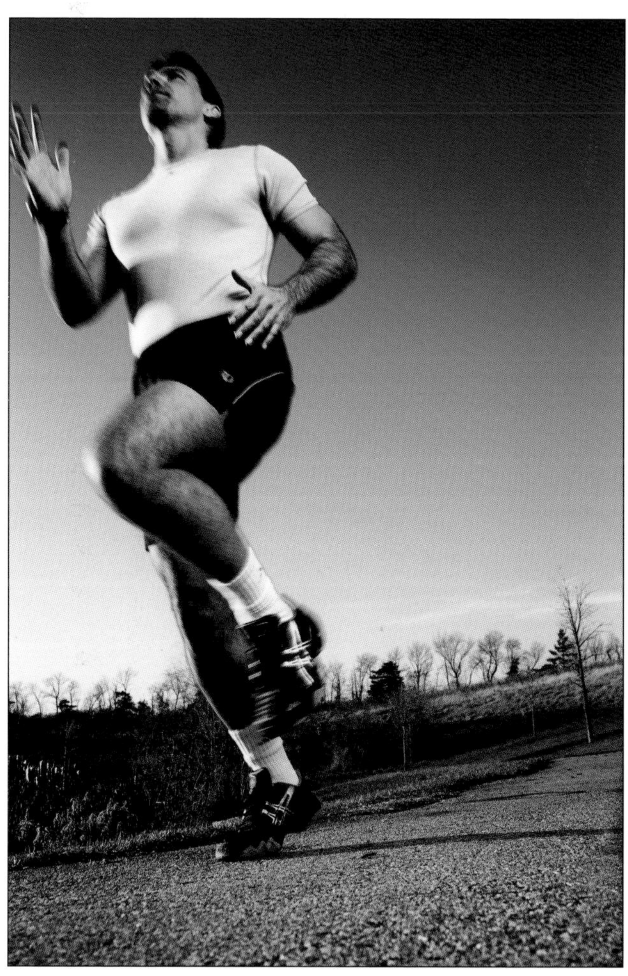

Interval training is repeated periods of higher-intensity exercise that lasts fifteen to thirty seconds. By placing these demands on the heart and the musculature, the body is being trained to withstand multiple three-minute intervals in the ring. Interval training is a great way to improve the anaerobic power and speed of a conditioned athlete.

Keep the interval training workouts short to start, and become familiar with how it feels to work at this higher intensity. The body produces more lactic acid as a by-product of the higher-intensity movement, and this may cause discomfort in the muscles, making you want to quit the activity. In addition the faster movements increase the chance of muscle strain or pulls. Your training heart-rate zone needs to be at 85 percent, with your effort between 90 to 100 percent.

Start with a ten-minute jog/run, then add a fifteen- to thirty-second sprint. Slow down the pace again to your initial speed for one to three minutes and repeat the cycle of sprinting and jogging for three to five times. Finish off with a slower-paced five- to ten-minute jog. Fast, short-distance running is a fun, challenging, and time-efficient way to exercise and build muscle power in the legs.

Track Sprints

Warm up with an easy run for ten to fifteen minutes, followed by some light stretches. Now, perform a series of sprints. Start your first sprint by gradually increasing your speed, aiming for foot push-off and turnover time to near maximum. Run 100 to 400 meters (109 to 437 yards) at sprint speed. Raise the knees high and pump the arms with each step. Keep the body tall and breathe deep into the abdomen. Once you have reached the desired distance, slow down and run easy for 400 to 800 meters (437 to 875 yards) to recover. Repeat 6 to 8 times. Always cool down with an easy five-minute recovery run after the final sprint. Strive for smooth quality sprints.

Timed Sprints

You can also incorporate timed sprints into your regular running route. These short speed sessions are best performed within a medium-length run.

Run for five minutes at your normal training pace to ensure that you are warmed up. As you begin your sprint, steadily increase your speed to near maximum over ten to thirty seconds. Resume running at your normal pace for two to three minutes to recover (or until you've returned to your training heart rate level). Now, perform your next sprint. In total, perform six to eight thirty-second sprints and finish up with a five- to ten-minute easy run.

Tips and Warnings

- Start off slightly slower than your maximum speed and gradually increase your pace with each new step.
- Adjust your pace or stop if you feel discomfort or pain.
- Ensure the running surface is flat and even.

Hill Training

Hill runs challenge your cardiovascular system and help develop quadriceps and calf muscle strength. Work at an intensity based on your current fitness level. Attack the hill not so fast that you have to stop halfway up, and not so slowly that you recover well before you reach the bottom. Training intensity can vary from 70 to 85 percent of your maximum heart rate during the uphill phase and recover to 60 percent in between hills. Perform hill training when you are well rested and not tired from the previous day's workout. Find a 200- to 400-yard hill that is fairly steep. Warm up for ten to twelve minutes with an easy run. Begin with four hill repeats, and increase by one each week to a maximum of twelve repeats. Always have at least two days to recover in between hill training.

There are specific techniques to use when running up and down hills. When running up lean slightly into the hill, using your arms and lifting your knees high, with rapid foot turn over. Keep your momentum forward and the level of physical effort relatively constant. Shift planting to the balls of the feet. Complete a run to the top of the hill. Turn around and walk or jog to the bottom, take a quick rest, and repeat. Find a hill with sure footing and a soft surface such as grass, or dirt.

Uphill Technique:

- Lean slightly into the hill, chest up.
- Shorten the stride, legs and arms working together.
- Shift foot plant to the balls of the feet.
- Keep your momentum forward, increasing effort as you approach the top.
- Run past the top.

Downhill Technique:

- Lean slightly forward, opening your stride.
- Let gravity grab you and pull you along.
- Focus on proper running technique.

Cardio-Conditioning Alternatives

If you want some variety in your training, traveling or weather conditions are prohibitive, there are a number of options available to train your cardio system.

A stationary bike is one great selection because it focuses on the development of the leg muscles. It may also be a good alternative to running if you are coming off of an injury, or if the weather conditions forbid outside activities.

To imitate the movement of running, treadmills are your best choice. The running motion on the treadmill is similar to running outside, but the push-off phase of the foot is different because the treadmill belt pulls the foot along. This produces a less-effective conditioning result. Although different from running on the ground, treadmills allow you to vary your running speed, can be inclined to imitate hill runs, and be formulated for a variety of different running programs.

Another great alternative is training on an elliptical trainer. You not only get a great aerobic workout, there is no stress on the joints. Elliptical trainers with dual action handlebars for the arms and foot pedals for the legs give a total body workout. The movement is smooth and strengthens the glutes, quadriceps, calves, and upper body muscles. When rehabilitating from an injury, the elliptical trainer provides a perfect alternative to maintain your cardiovascular fitness levels. It is also challenging for the seasoned athlete.

Boxers jump rope as part of their fitness training. The jump rope is a great alternative to maintain and improve overall aerobic conditioning when traveling.

Flexibility and Stretching

It is important to maintain good flexibility throughout your life. Flexibility decreases with the aging process, resulting in joint stiffness, tight muscle, decreased range of motion, and poor posture. Stretching helps to keep the body limber, making activity and movement easier.

For each joint area, the muscles, tendons, ligaments, and bone-on-bone connections are able to achieve a certain degree of movement. This is known as the range of motion. And for each movement, activity, or sport there is an optimal range of motion required to produce the desired outcome. Sports such as gymnastics will require a far greater range of motion at the hip joint

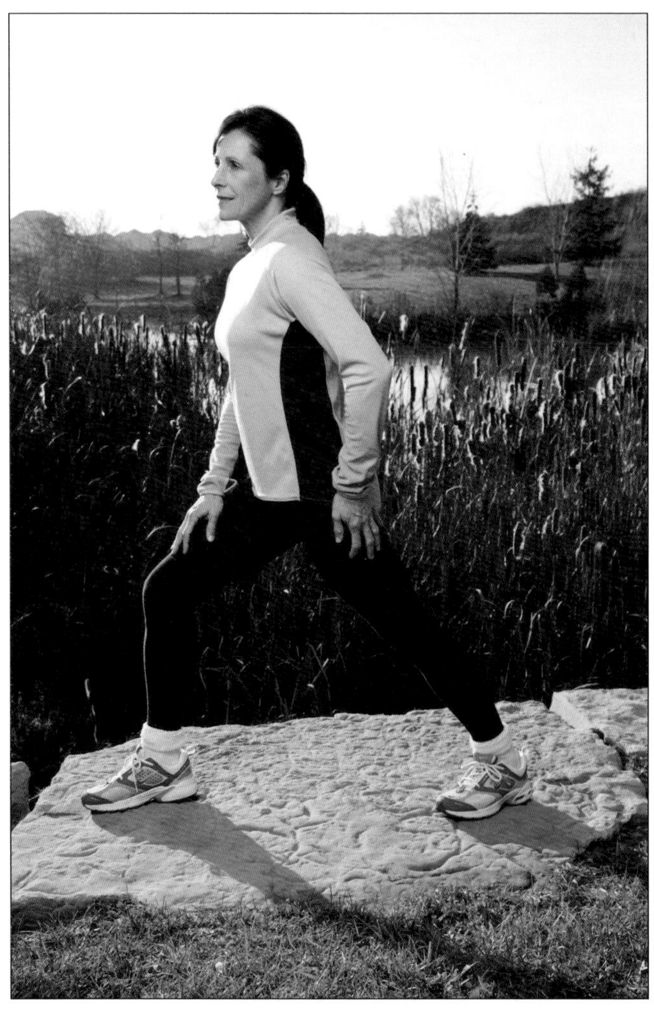

and through the muscles of the legs, whereas activities such as running or boxing will require less in these areas.

Reduced flexibility of the muscles and the joint areas can lead to a number of problems both during training and during normal daily activity. The result of poor flexibility is injury, pain, and discomfort. There must always be a balance in the strength of a muscle and its extensibility. Muscular imbalance can be caused by both sports-specific demands, making some muscle too tight and inflexible, and also by poor postural habits. A strong muscle that is pliable and limber withstands stress from activity better than a strong, rigid, inflexible muscle. Poor posture may cause muscles to be tightened and shortened, creating problems in associated joints. For example, extensive running without stretching afterwards may reduce the flexibility at the hip joint, reducing the length of the hip flexor muscles. This overpowers a weak lower back and causes pain, possibly generating down into the back of the legs. By stretching out the hip flexor area and strengthening the lower back and abdominal area, the pain and muscle imbalance can be corrected. Daily stretching promotes the proper alignment of the muscle tissue, lengthening out muscles that are tight, inflexible, and overused. As the range of motion is increased at the joint area, performance can be optimized, greatly reducing the risk of injury.

The degree to which you are flexible is specific to each individual. Tendon and ligament length, genetics, the elasticity within the muscle tissue, and lifestyle are all determinants of the degree to which you can stretch. Stretch whenever your muscles feel tight, and take it through an optimal range of motion. There are two different types of stretches: static and dynamic. When performing a static stretch, you lengthen and hold the muscle for a specified amount of time. It is a very controlled stretch with very little visible movement. A dynamic stretch elongates the muscle to a certain length while moving. This type of stretch is still very controlled, but visible movement does occur while the muscle is being stretched. Of course, there is a higher risk of tearing muscle fibers when performing dynamic stretches, and care must be taken to be in control and not bounce or jar into a position (ballistic stretch).

A pre-activity stretch or warm-up stretch is an easy stretch aimed at taking the muscle and joints through a full range of motion, which imitates the movements of the activity to follow. It is often a dynamic stretch, which increases the blood flow to the working muscles. The muscles are being prepared for activity and for initiating neuromuscular coordination. This stretch is held for ten to fifteen seconds, reducing muscle tightness. The purpose is not to increase the muscle in total length, but just to warm up the area.

The post-activity stretch is aimed at relaxing and lengthening the working muscle to normal length. After the workout, the body and muscle temperature is elevated, and the risk of tearing a muscle fiber or the connective tissue is reduced. This is the time to work on improving your flexibility and lengthening the muscle beyond what is normal to you. Stretching will also promote the removal of workout waste by-products (like lactic acid) from the muscles and provide new nutrients to rebuild the muscle tissue. Slow, static stretching is effective in reducing the localized muscle soreness after exercising, and it assists in increasing the amounts and the quality of synovial fluid available at the joint areas. This allows freer movement and easier at the bone-on-bone connections. A post-activity stretch is held for at least fifteen to forty seconds, holding the stretch at a point where mild tension is felt, relaxing and then moving a fraction further into the stretch.

Remember that stretching is not competitive and should be performed in a relaxed environment. It has a way of promoting a sense of well-being and will increase your awareness of your body and musculature.

Do not bounce into a stretch. Using force will not increase the flexibility; it only causes the stretch reflex impulse to contract the muscle fibers, resulting in microscopic tearing of the muscle fibers. This in turn reduces the elasticity of the muscle, resulting in soreness and tightness. Also, do not over-stretch. It is far better to under-stretch than over-stretch a muscle. Try to find the point where you feel the stretch and are able to relax at the same time. Relaxation of the muscle tissue and performing the stretches are the two most important factors in improving your flexibility. By stretching on a regular basis, improvements in muscle length are very noticeable and beneficial to performance.

Stretching Exercises

Standing Quadricep/Hip Flexor Stretch

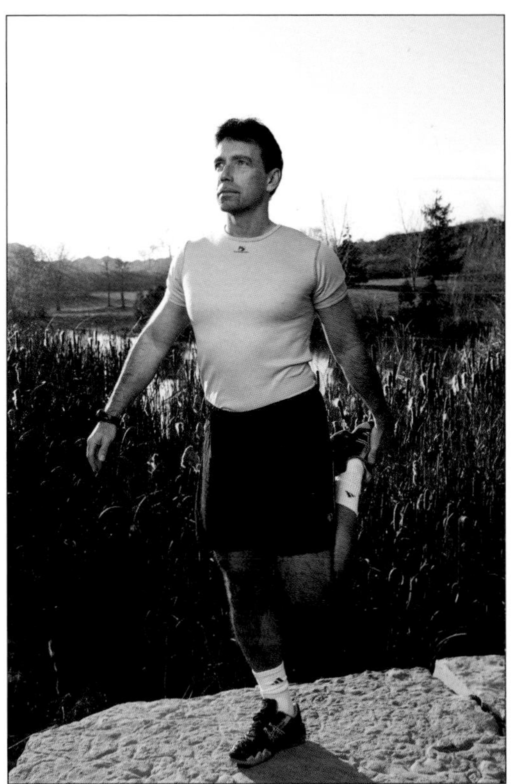

Stand on one leg. Lift one leg back, keeping the knees together, and hold onto the ankle or lower leg with the arm on the same side. Stand tall, with the torso held tight and pull the heel up towards the buttocks. You should feel a slight stretch in the front of the leg or quadriceps muscle. To stretch the hip flexor, press the hips forward while keeping the knees together and bending the supporting leg slightly. Hold from ten to thirty seconds and repeat. Perform and repeat several times with each leg.

Standing Calf/Achilles Stretch

Stand with one leg forward and one leg back. With both feet facing straight forward, bend the front leg and shift the body towards the front foot. Keep the back heel on the floor. You will feel a stretch in the center of the calf muscle. To stretch the achilles tendon and the lower part of the calf, bend the back knee slightly, shift the body weight backward a little, and keep the back heel on the floor. Hold from ten to thirty seconds and repeat. Perform five to seven times on each side.

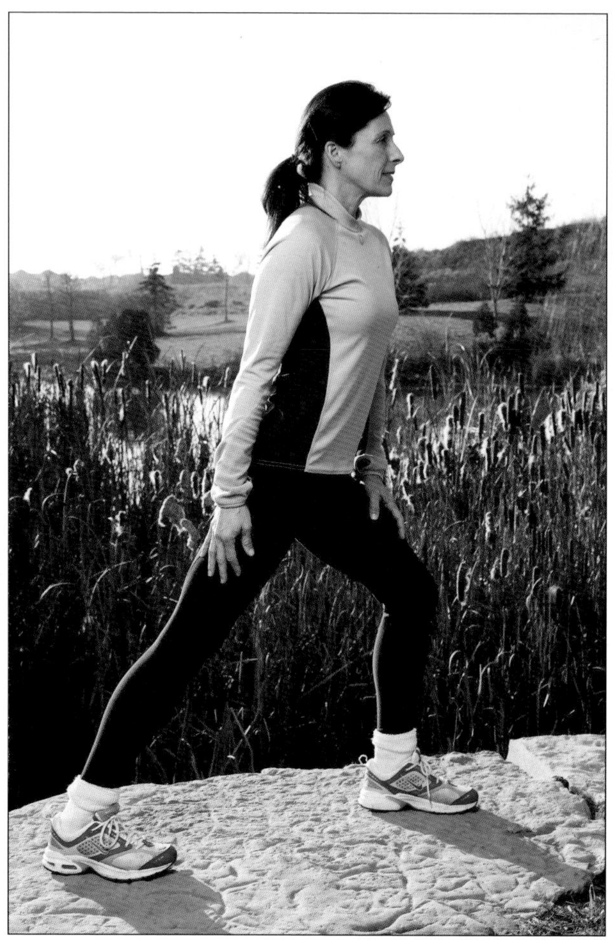

Seated Hamstring Stretch

Sitting on the floor comfortably, one leg extended and the other bent in towards the body and on the floor. Flex the foot of the extended leg and bend the body forward from the hips, keeping the back as flat as possible. Reach forward only to the point where you are still relaxed and feel the stretch or tension at the back of the extended leg. Release and repeat. Perform five to seven times with each leg.

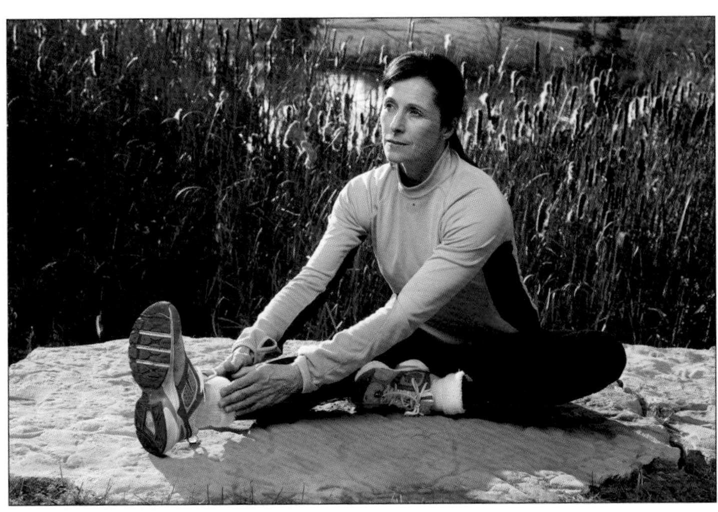

Supine Hamstring Stretch

Lie on your back, one leg bent with the foot on the ground. Hold the extended leg with your hands and pull towards your chest until the first tension is felt in

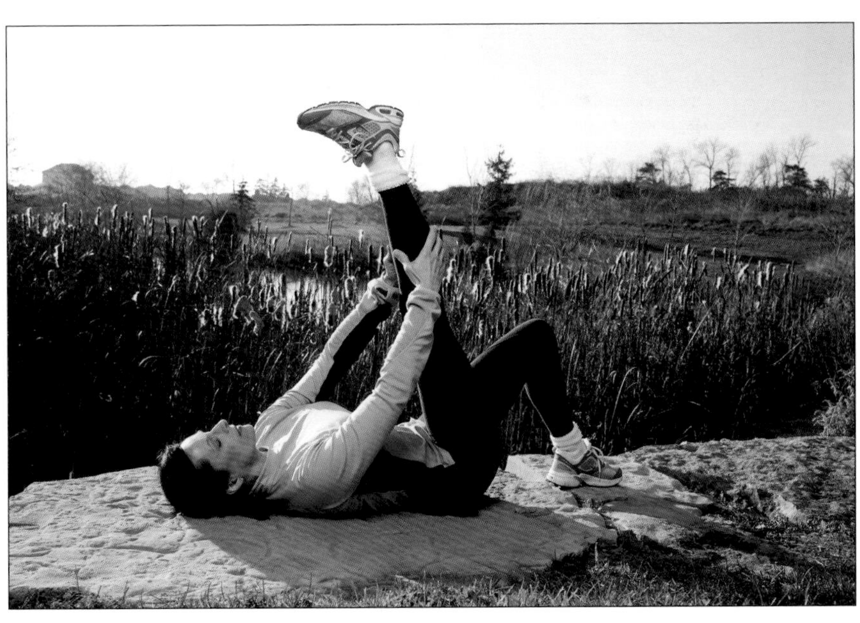

the hamstring muscle. Maintain this position until the muscle relaxes and the tension disappears, and then release. Perform five to seven times with each leg.

Seated Hip Stretch

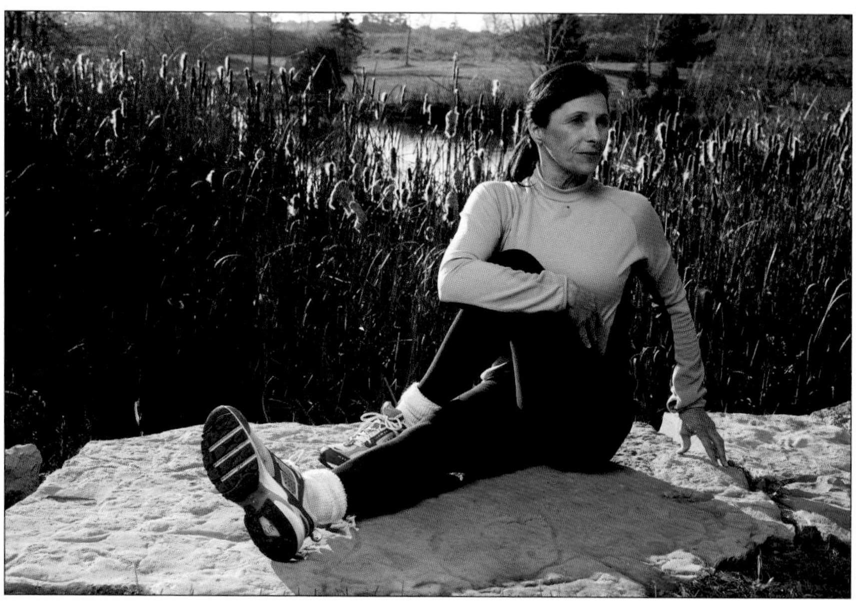

Sitting on the floor, one leg extended in front and the other bent at the knee, foot on the outside of the extended leg. Pull the knee in towards the opposite shoulder and close to the body. Rotate the upper body looking over the back shoulder. Sit tall and hold the stretch. Release and repeat three to five times with each leg.

Upper Back Stretch

Sit or stand with the arms extended in front of the body, and hold the hands together with the palms facing away from the body. Press the hands and arms forward from the shoulder region allowing the back to round. You should feel the stretch throughout the upper back. Hold for ten to thirty seconds, and repeat several times.

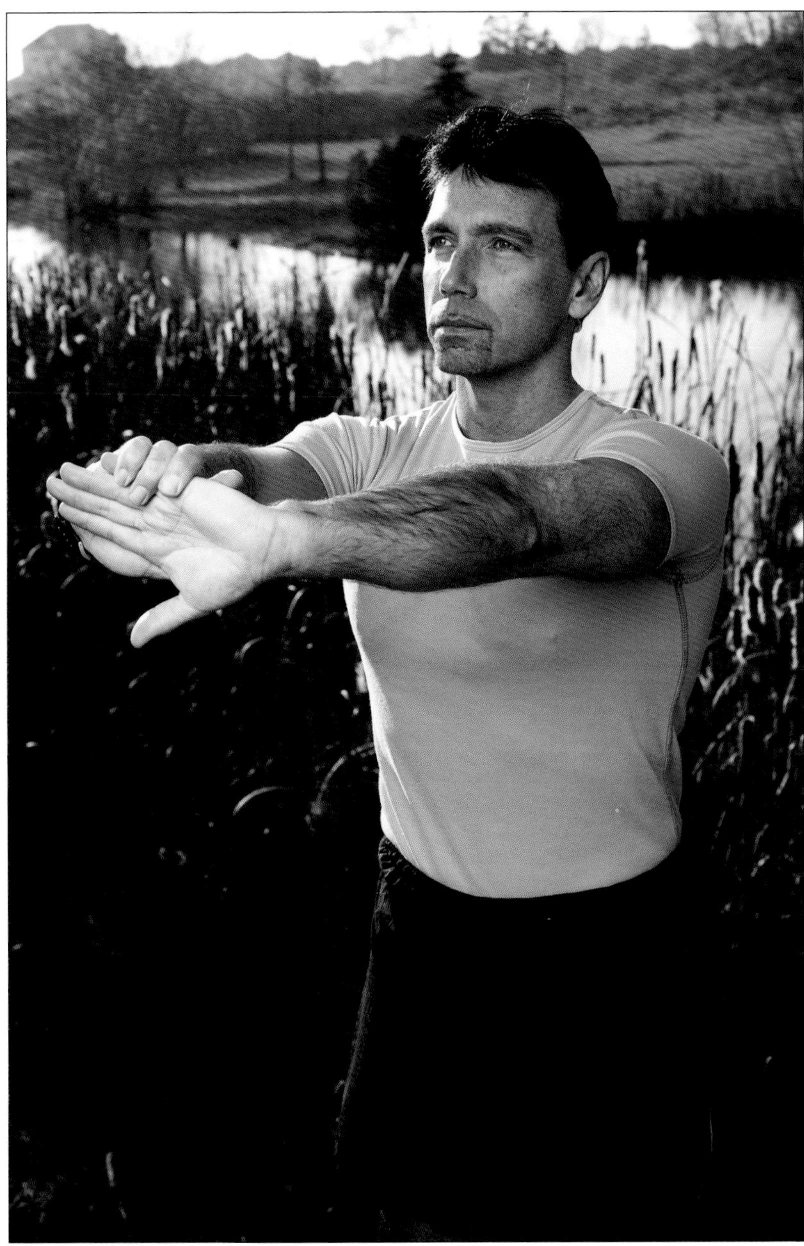

Chest and Shoulder Stretch

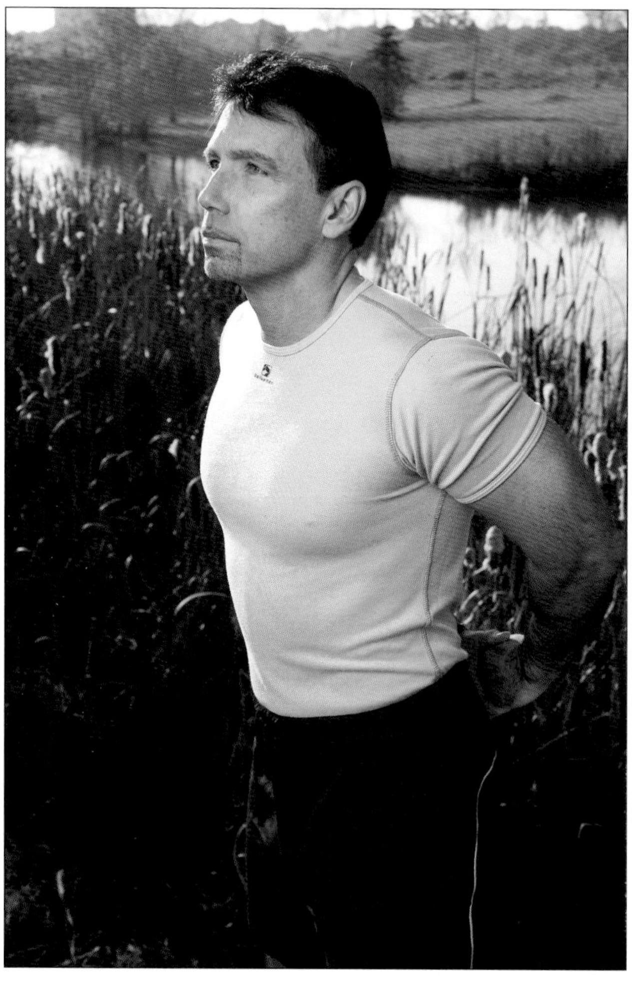

Stand tall, knees relaxed, abdominal muscles tight, arms extended behind the back, and the fingers interlaced. Straighten the arms by rotating the elbows inward, then lift the arms up behind you slightly, stretching through the shoulders, chest, and arms. Hold the stretch for five to fifteen seconds, and repeat several times.

Shoulder and Middle of Upper Back Stretch

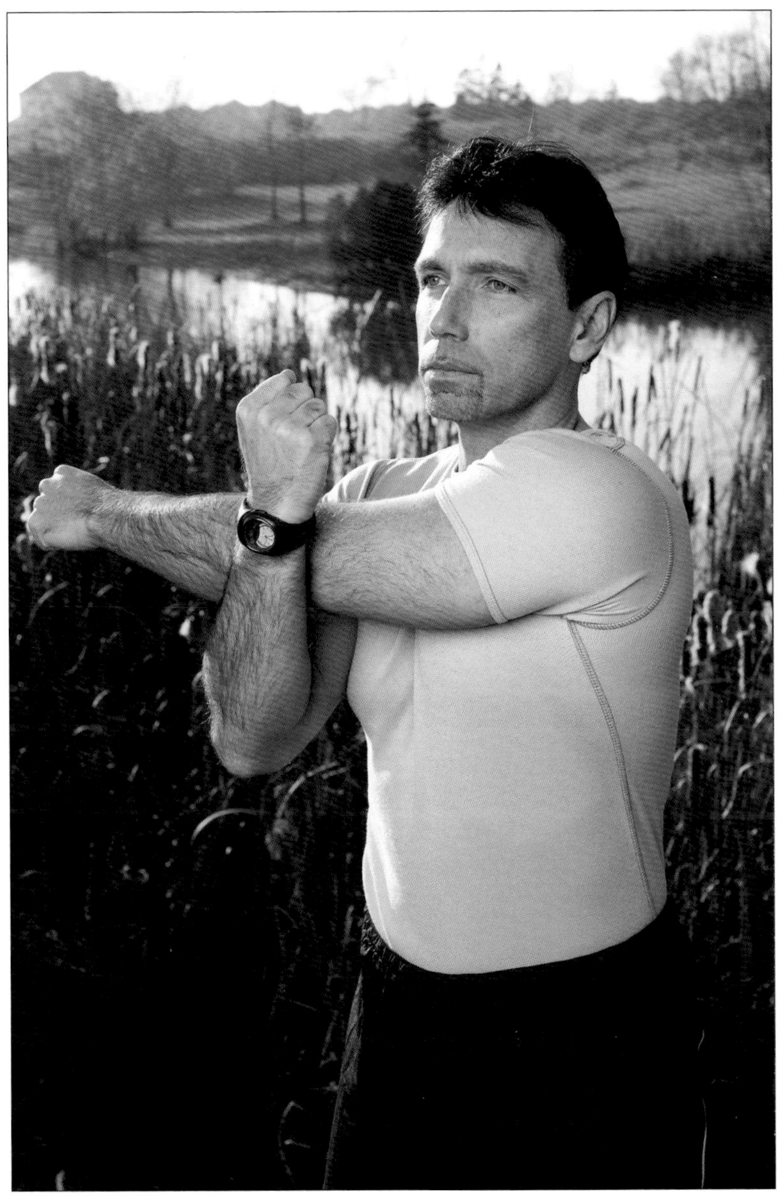

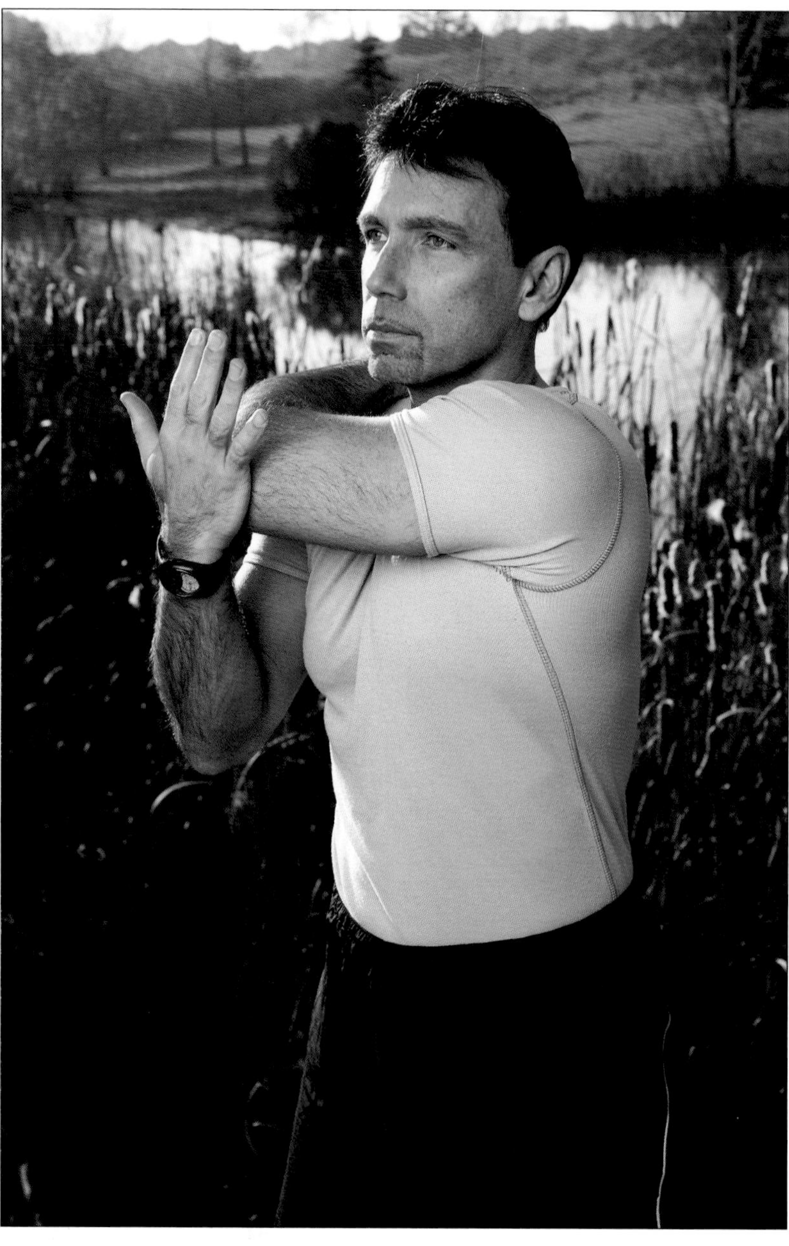

Stand or sit with one arm crossed in front of the body. Hold onto this arm, keeping it straight. Gently press across the chest to the opposite shoulder, stretching the middle of the upper back. To stretch more of the shoulder area, bend the arm at the elbow, and press across the chest. Hold each stretch for five to fifteen seconds, and repeat several times.

Triceps and Shoulder Stretch

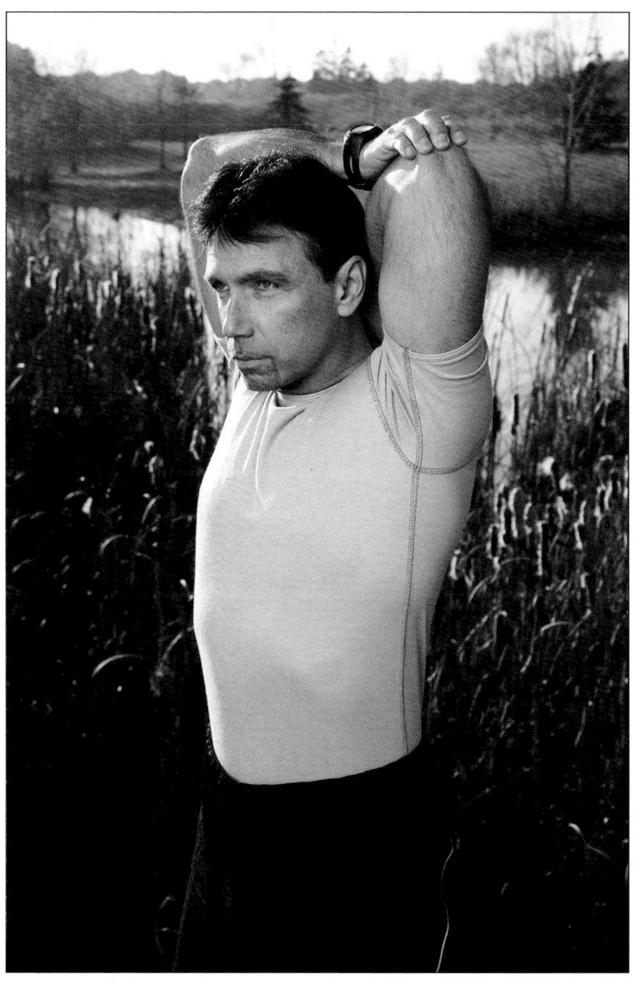

Stand or sit tall with the head facing forward and both arms held overhead. Hold onto one elbow with the opposite hand, and gently press the other hand down the center of the back. Hold for ten to fifteen seconds, and repeat several times.

Reminders for Stretching:

- Before a run, take the muscles through an optimal range of motion with no tension exerted on the muscles. After a run, stretch all the working muscles allowing them to return to their resting length.
- Isolate the muscle group. Do not place any stress on the joints.
- Find zero tension on the muscle. This is your starting point.
- Perform the stretch finding the first gentle tension on the muscle. Hold this steady position.
- Hold the stretch long enough to allow the tension to disappear and the muscle to relax.

Muscle Conditioning

9

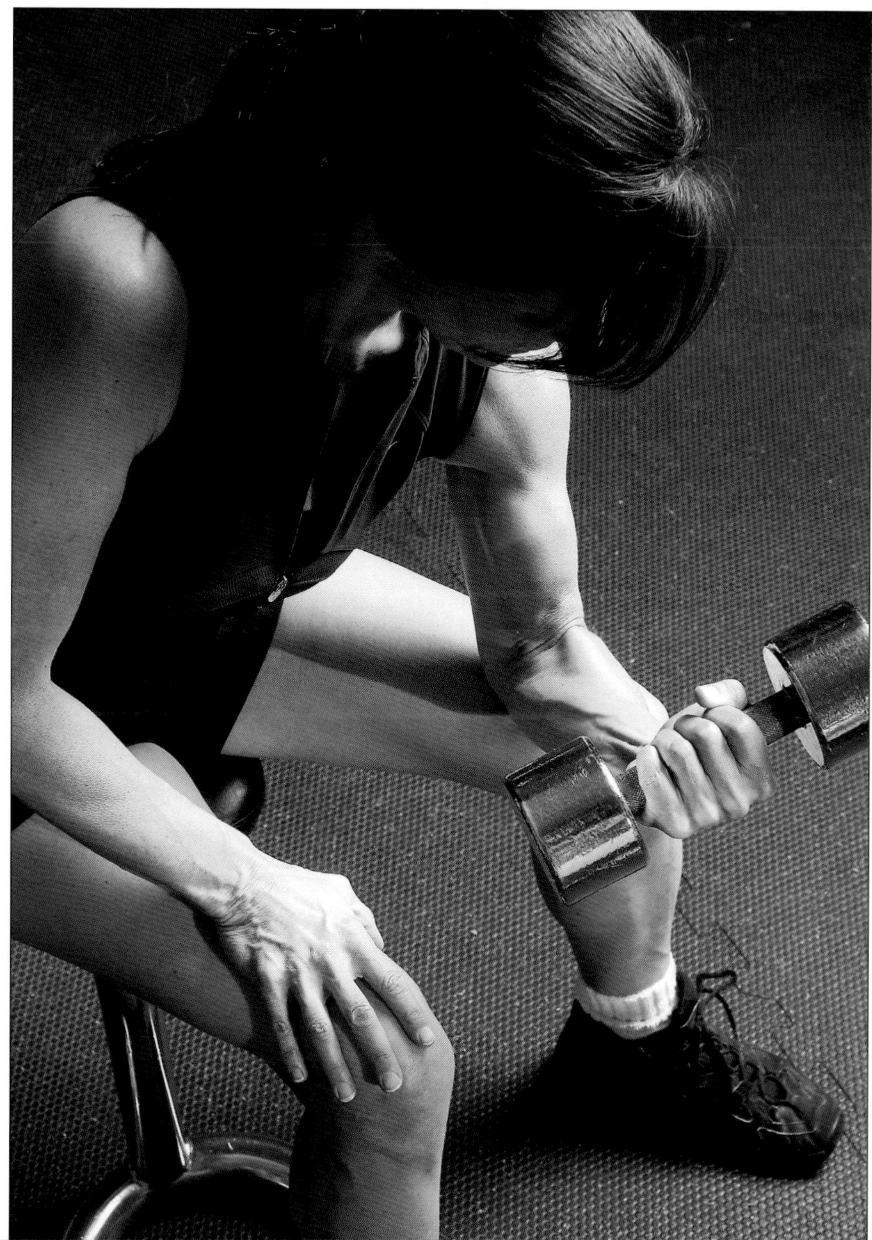

At one time, weight training was not part of the boxer's workout regimen. It was believed that weight training would produce a muscle-bound, slower-moving boxer in the ring, and that bag work, roadwork, and sparring were sufficient training to increase speed and punching power. But, as some of the more recent boxers have discovered, weight training better prepares you for the battle in the ring. It puts power into the punches and stability into the stance, and it reduces the occurrences of joint and muscle injuries. Weight training increases overall stamina, punching and foot speed, and lean body mass, and it develops the torso to be able to absorb body punches. Professional boxers of the modern era like Oscar Del La Hoya, Jermain Taylor, and Floyd Mayweather Jr., believe that strength training is essential to the whole training package, complementing the overall outcome.

Muscles give the body form. They produce movement by receiving and responding to orders from the brain and central nervous system. Each one of us is in control of sending information to the muscle fibers, so that the muscles may produce movement. With specific training, the muscles learn how to respond faster and more efficiently and effectively to specific demands. With continual repetition of a movement, the muscle fiber instinctively performs the movement requested. When we perform and demand the very best and the very extreme from each movement, the muscle fiber increases in strength and circumference with an improved outcome—a greater muscle mass.

The Muscle Conditioning Program

The most efficient and positive method to improve strength and develop muscle tissue is to weight train. Weight training is recognized as an important facet of total fitness and is incorporated into the Old School Boxing Workout twice a week. Day three and day six of the program are spent on training a variety of muscles specific to improving boxing movements.

You may wonder why this program suggests training with weights only twice a week when traditionally bodybuilders train six days a week. Bodybuilders train specific muscle groups twice a week and will have three different workouts, giving six workout days. Time is spent training very specific muscle groups in each session, and the different muscle groups are worked only twice a week. In the Old School Boxing Workout, all the muscle groups are worked in each weight training session twice per week. The emphasis is on using weight training to supplement the overall workout program, promoting improved capabilities for the boxing workout. The program encourages muscular strength and endurance, which in turn provides the basis for stronger and more powerful punches. Improvements in speed, technique, agility and response time will result from lifting weights.

Traditionally, when training with weights, eight to twelve repetitions of an exercise are performed, and this is repeated three times. Our goal is to provide a program that will give you strength gains in the least amount of time. The method of weight training used here will be based on lifting a specified weight a maximum of ten times in the second set of the exercise routine, when the eleventh lift cannot be completed. This ten-rep maximum is the basis for setting the weight used in the first set and third sets.

In the first set, the goal is to lift the weight more than ten times (around twelve reps). This is usually around 80 percent of the weight used for the ten-rep max. In the second set, the weight is increased, so that the muscle will fatigue at ten reps. In the third set, the weight is reduced to the same weight as used in the first set, and the weight is lifted as many times as possible until total muscle failure occurs.

If you have trained with weights previously, it should be easy to determine your ten-rep max. If you are new to weight training, start with a lighter weight, perhaps lifting the weight twelve to fourteen repetitions. If you are able to complete eleven reps or more, then you know you will need a heavier weight for the next set. If, on the other hand, you cannot complete a set of ten reps, the weight is too heavy, and for the next set the poundage should be reduced. It may take two or three workouts (one to two weeks), to determine your exact ten-rep max. It is always better to find your ten-rep max by lifting a lighter weight and placing stress on the muscle fiber by increasing the number of repetitions than by trying to lift a weight that you cannot even push eight times. The risk of injury increases, especially to the connecting tissues (ligaments and tendons).

By causing the muscle to go to failure (unable to perform the lift), stress or an overload has been placed on the muscle fibers. The waste material, lactic acid, inhibits the muscle contractile system to respond to the requested work. It will take the lactic acid thirty to forty-five seconds to break up, and then the exercise should be repeated. Muscles adapt to the added weight/stress and will perform at a greater weight after they have repaired (usually twenty-four to forty-eight hours).

First set: 80 percent of ten-rep max (twelve to fourteen reps)
Second set: 100 percent of ten-rep max (ten reps)
Third set: 80 percent of ten-rep max (repetitions to fatigue)

Order of Exercises

The exercises should be performed in the order that they are listed, from the largest muscle group to the smallest ones. It is important to work the larger muscles first because the smaller muscles are required for stability. The smaller muscle is the weak link. When the larger muscles are worked, the smaller muscles assist in the movement for the larger muscles.

For example, the bench press requires the use of the chest muscles, and the triceps muscle assists in the lifting movement. If the triceps are fatigued, the pectoral muscles will not execute the movement properly and inhibit the development of the chest.

Weight Equipment

We have included free weights, weight machines, and the medicine ball in the program. Free weights are often the preferred option for weight lifting because it is easy to adapt and alter exercises. Factors like balance, increased range of movement, symmetrical development, muscle uniformity, and control are better satisfied with the use of free weights over machines. When using free weights, it is best to work with a partner and have him or her spot or assist you when performing the exercise. This is especially important with high-risk exercises, when the weight has the potential of falling on the lifter. Because this workout includes lifting a weight to a ten-rep max in order to produce muscle failure, a spotter should be available to assist with the weight, if needed. If a spotter is not available, and you are performing a high-risk exercise, (e.g., the bench press), the weight being lifted and/or the number of repetitions being performed should be reduced. The muscle should not be taken to failure.

The use of weight machines with cable systems or self-spotting devices allows you to perform an exercise to muscle failure if you are working out on your own. The weight equipment (free or machines) at any gym should be studied, and choices should be made according to availability of a spotting partner, the fit of the machine to your body frame, and the hopeful outcome of the exercise.

Body position, the execution of the exercise, and breathing are important elements to remember when lifting. Exhale on effort, or when pressing the weight away from the starting position, and inhale on relaxation, or when returning the weight back to the starting position. Find a comfortable rate of execution. It should not be too quick because the momentum of the weight, not your muscle power, will be carrying the limb to the end position. Try to take the weight through the full range of motion, engaging a broad array of muscle fibers. Move the weight from the starting position in a controlled manner, pause, and then go back again to the finish position. The movement is smooth and controlled. It is important to keep the body in the correct position as shown in the photographs. The core is held tight, and all posture and supporting muscle are in alignment, so that the exercise may be executed correctly. This also reduces chance of injury in the working muscle and supports muscles and joint regions.

Some Considerations

The weight that you are able to lift may vary from workout to workout. Some days you may feel stronger and be able to press more weight; other days you may feel fatigued before you even start. Extraneous conditions such as health and personal commitments can influence your workout capabilities. A reduced ability in lifting weights is often noticed during your first set. If during your first set you struggled to get ten reps or did not even reach that number, reduce the weight for the second set. Do not forgo your workout; try to keep your schedule; just reduce the intensity of the workout.

Exercises With Weights

A combination of free weight and machine exercises have been chosen for this program. Perform the exercises in the following order:

<u>Incline Dumbbell Bench Press</u>

Free weights or weight machine
Targeted area: pectoralis major, and serratus anterior

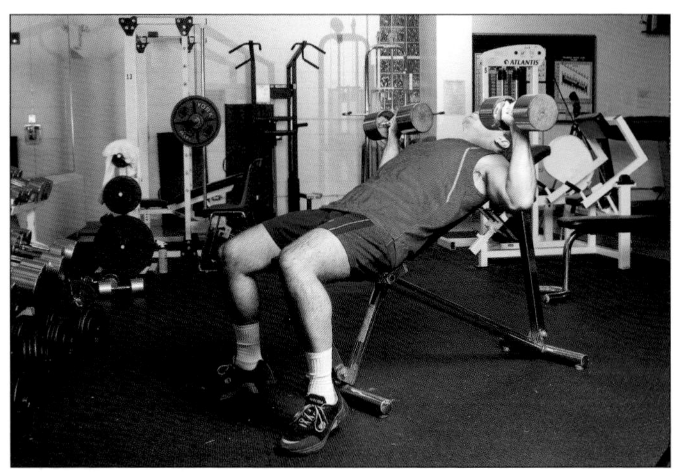

Dumbbell bench press–start

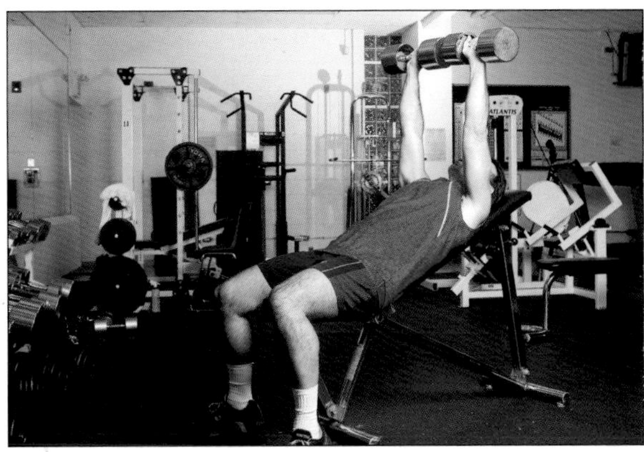

Dumbbell bench press–finish

Lie on your back on an inclined flat bench, set at an angle less than 60 degrees. Elbows bent at a right angle with respect to the upper arm, hold the dumbbells in an overhand grip, inhale and press the weights away from the chest, extending the arms until the weights touch softly. Exhale and slowly lower the weights towards the chest.

Lat Pull-Down

Weight machine
Targeted area: latissimus dorsi and teres major

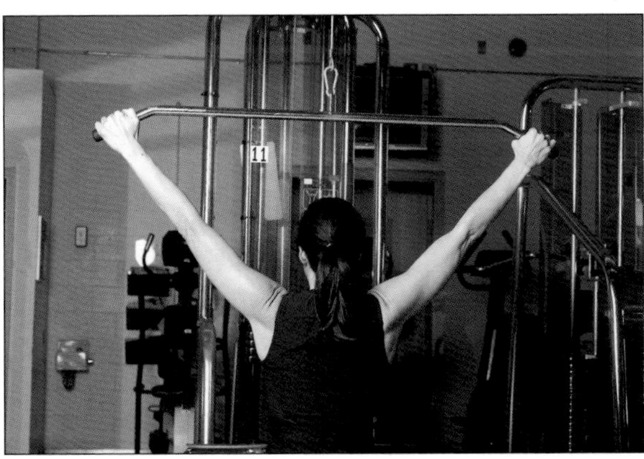

Lat pull-down–start

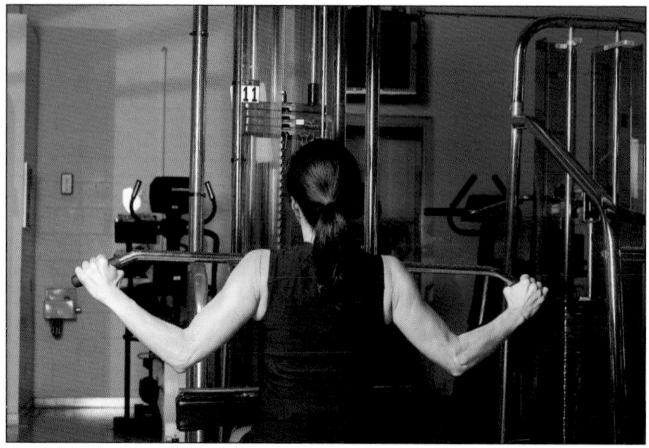

Lat pull-down–finish

Sit facing the weight machine. Hold the bar in an overhand wide grip, arms extended. Sit tall, leaning slightly back, chest lifted forward and knees steadied under the leg pads. Inhale and pull the bar down on an angle towards the upper chest. Squeeze the shoulder blades together by bringing the elbows back as you pull through. Pause and exhale, returning the bar to the starting position slowly and with control.

Seated Pec Deck

Weight Machine
Targeted area: pectoralis major and serratus anterior

Sit with the arms out at right angles (bent up at the elbows) at shoulder level and the forearms placed on the pads of the weight machine. Keep the back straight, shoulders relaxed, and look straight ahead. Bring the arms together, contracting the center of the chest and pulling from the elbow area until the pads come together. Pause and return the pads to the starting position. Exhale as the arms are bought together, and inhale as the arms open up towards toward the sides.

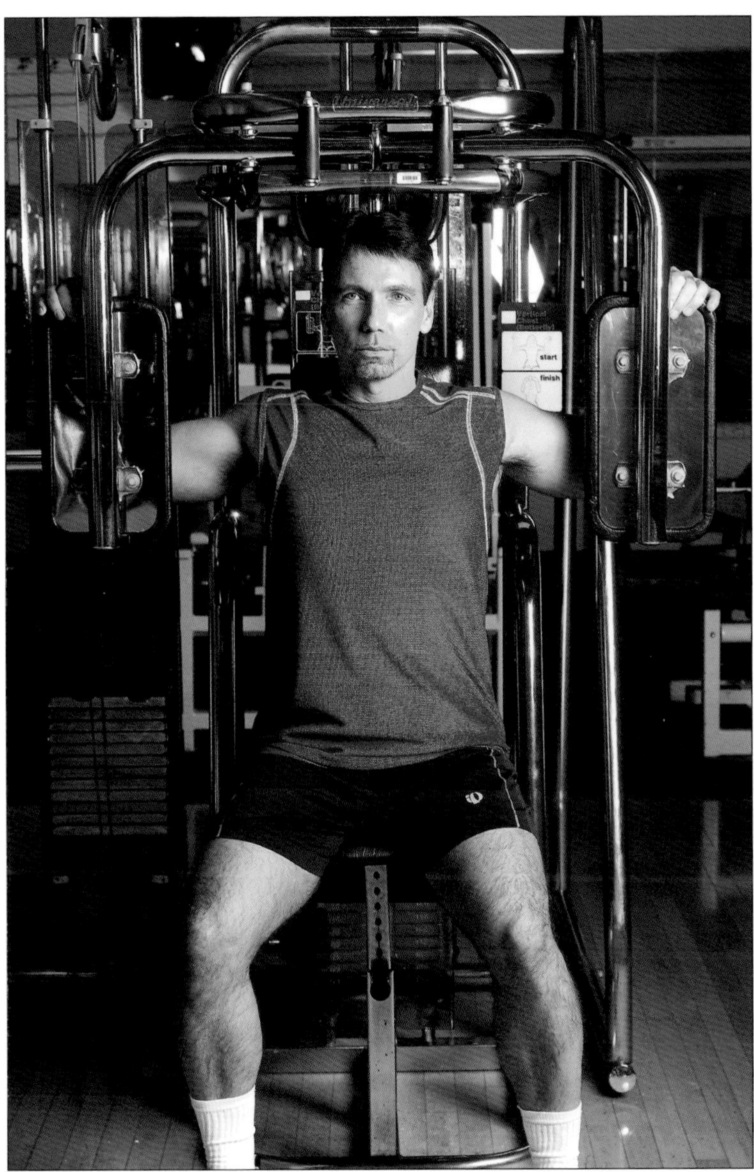

Seated pec deck–start

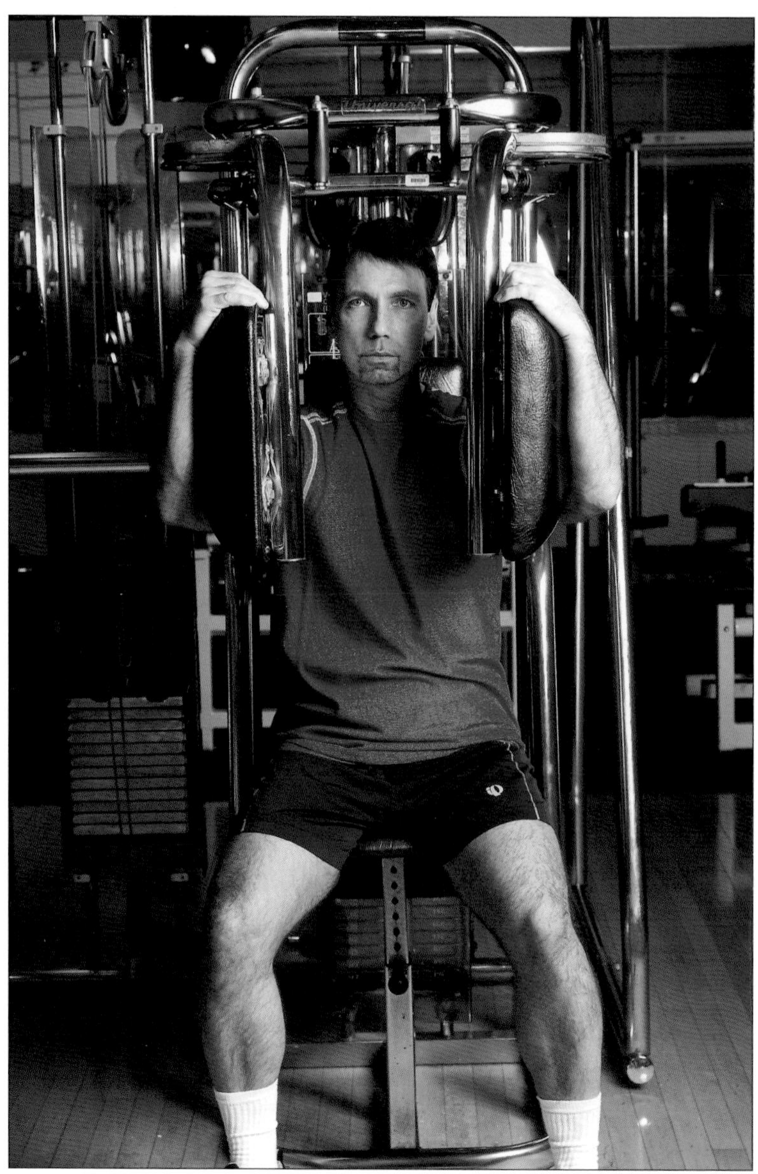

Seated pec deck–finish

Bent Over Dumbbell Row

Free weights

Targeted area: latissimus dorsi and rhomboideus

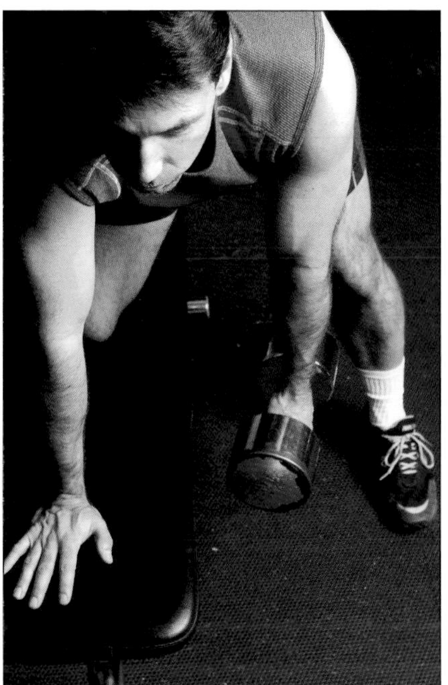

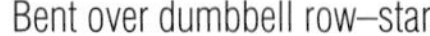

Bent over dumbbell row–start

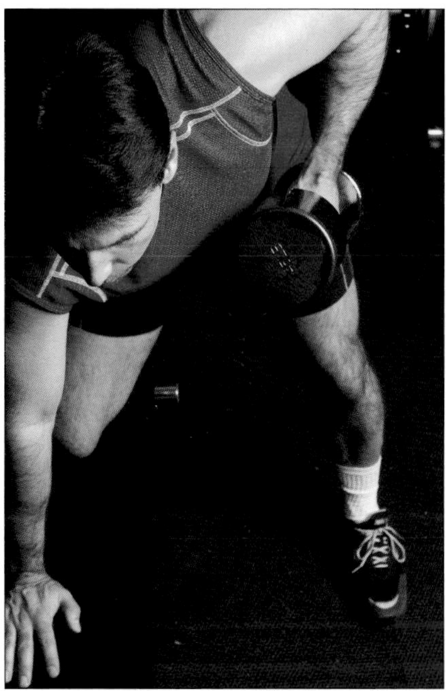

Bent over dumbbell row–finish

Place one knee on a flat bench. Lean forward with the body, hold the weight in one hand, and place the other hand forward on the flat bench for torso support. Keep the back flat and the head in line with it. Hold the weight in an overhand grip (knuckles forward) with the arm extended straight under the shoulder. Bring the shoulder blade toward the centerline of the body, then lift the elbow straight up toward the ceiling. The hand will rotate slightly with the knuckles facing out. There can also be a slight rotation of the body as the weight reaches shoulder height. Pause and slowly return the weight to the starting position. Ensure that the weight is lowered directly under the shoulder and not toward the back foot. Inhale as the weight is raised and exhale as the weight is lowered. Repeat with the other arm.

Side and Front Arm Raises

Free Weights
Targeted area: anterior/medial deltoid

Stand with feet hip-width apart and the knees relaxed. Hold the torso tight, and initiate all movement from the shoulder region. To perform side arm raises, extend the arms at the sides of the body and hold the weights with the knuckles facing out. Raise the arms up to shoulder height laterally (out to the side of the body). Pause and then lower the arms slowly to the starting position. To perform front arm raises, extend the arms in front of the body, knuckles facing front. Raise straight forward, shoulder height only, pause, and then lower the arms slowly to the starting position.

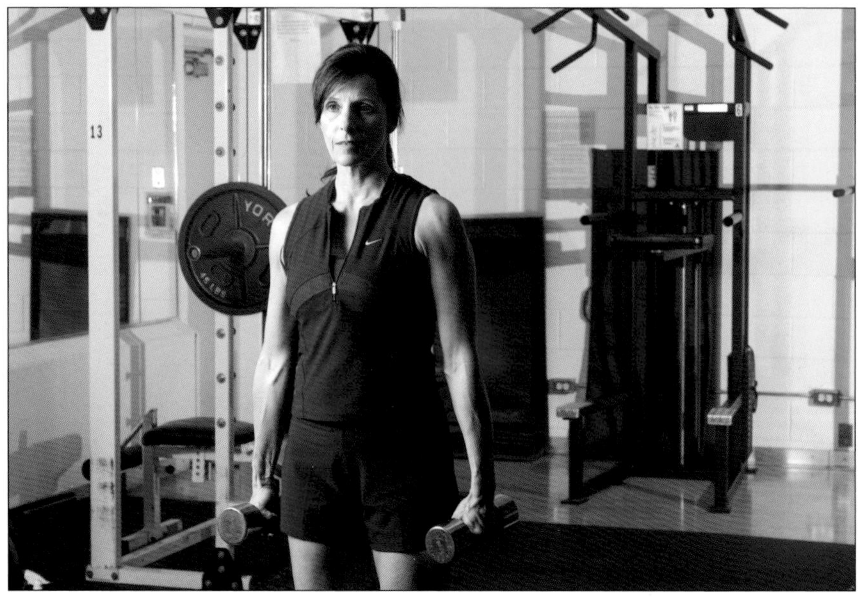

Side arm raise–start

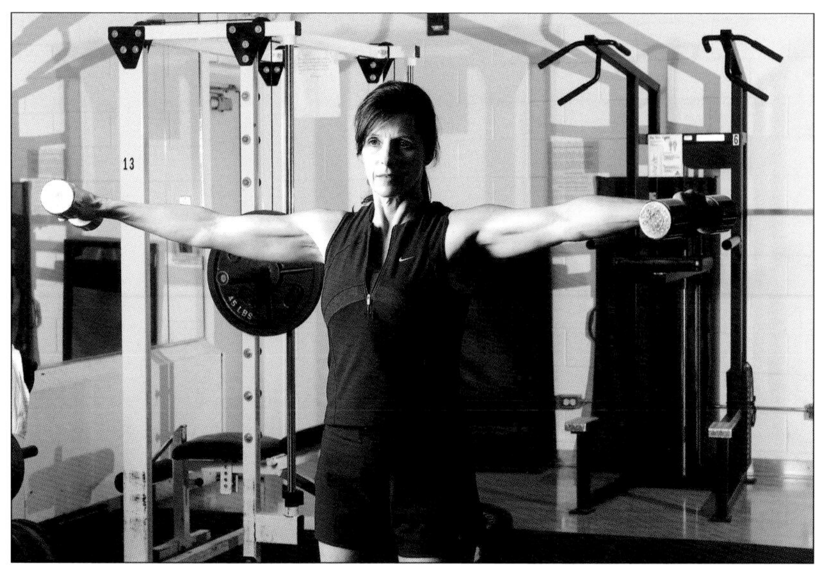

Side arm raise–finish

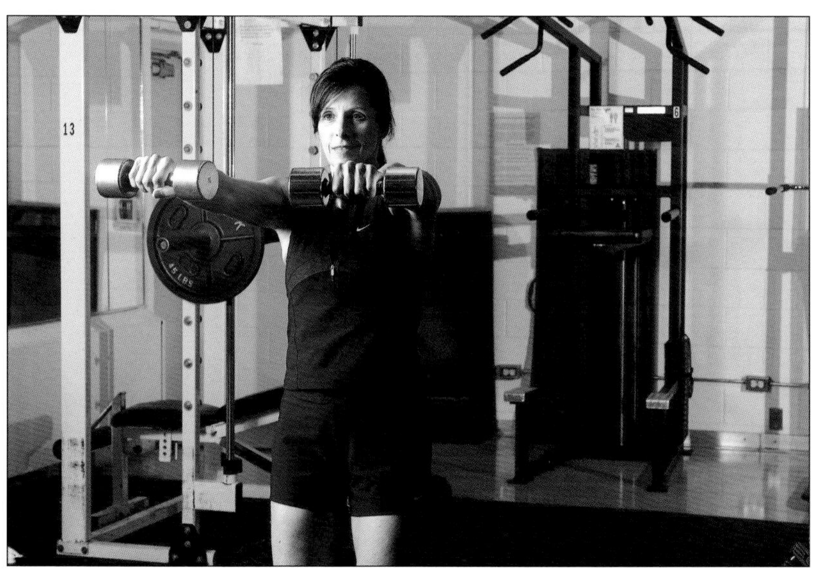

Front arm raise

Biceps Curl

Free Weights

Targeted area: biceps brachii

Stand with feet hip-width apart, the abdominals held tight, and the arms slightly bent at the elbow to maintain tension on the muscle. Extend the arms close to the sides of the body. Hold the weights in an underhand grip, knuckles facing either forward or in towards the body. Keeping the torso

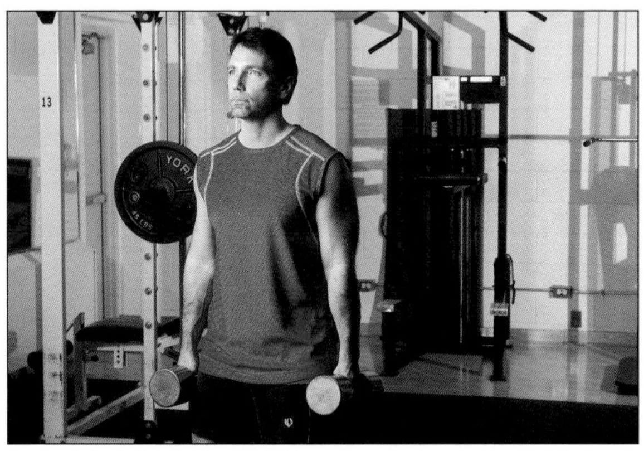

Biceps curl–start

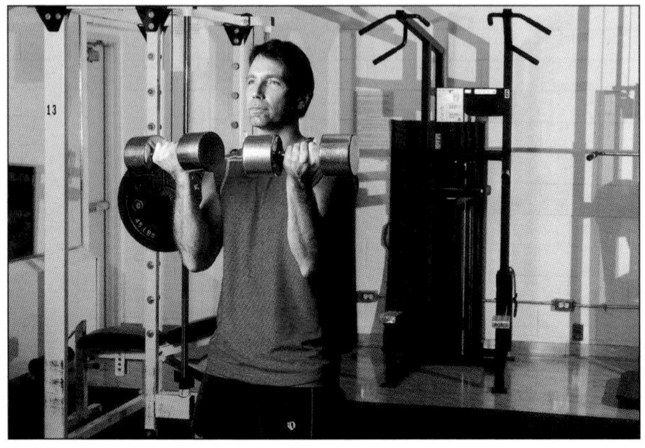

Biceps curl–finish

strong and the elbows close to the body. Raise the weights up towards the chest area. Pause at the top and lower the weights to the starting position, stopping in front of the thighs.

Triceps Pull-Down

Weight Machine

Targeted area: triceps brachii, teres major, and teres minor

Stand facing the machine. Hold the bar with both hands in an overhand close grip at chest level. Place the feet slightly closer than hip-width apart, with the knees relaxed and the torso tight. Keep the elbows close to the body and press the bar down toward the upper thighs until the arms are extended. Pause and slowly return the bar to the starting position, keeping the elbows at the sides of the body. Exhale as you press the bar down, and inhale as you release the bar.

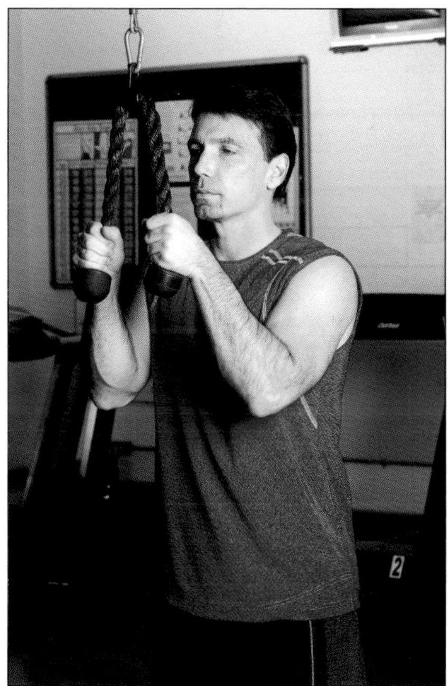

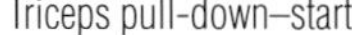

Triceps pull-down–start

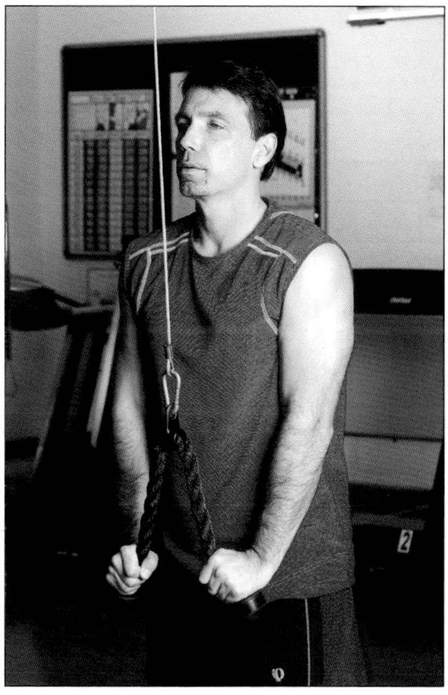

Triceps pull-down–finish

Leg Extension

Weight Machine

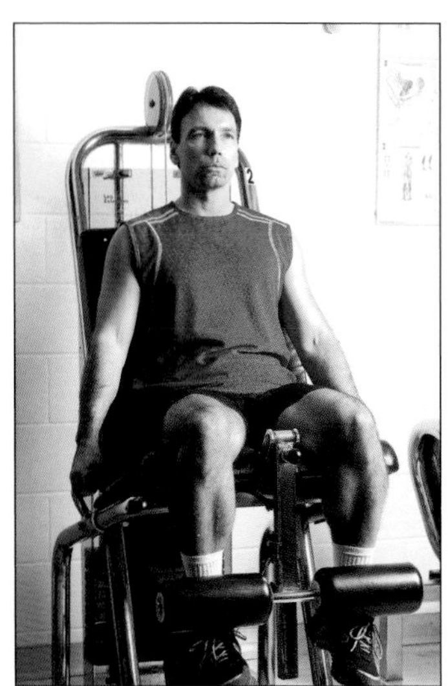

Leg extension–start

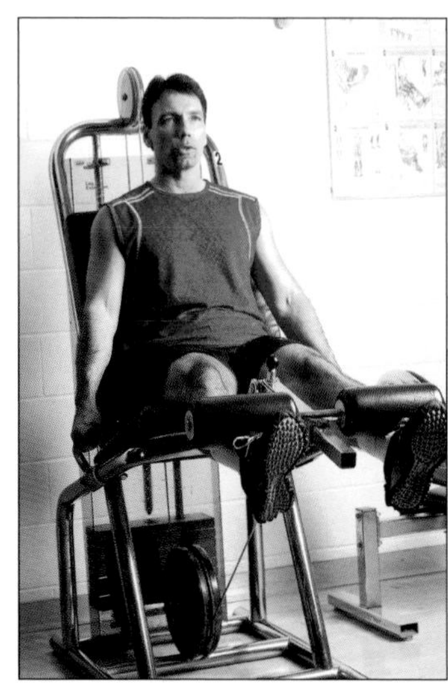

Leg extension–finish

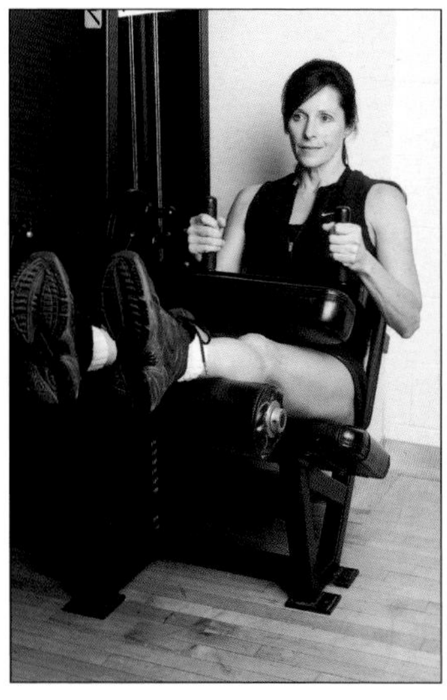

Seated hamstring curl–start

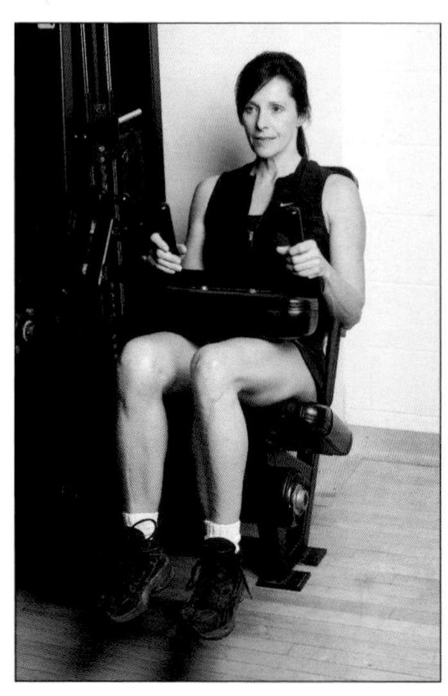

Seated hamstring curl–finish

Targeted area: quadriceps, rectus femoris, vastus medialis, lateralis, and intermedius

Sit tall on the bench, with the back supported and the thighs fully on the bench. Contract the quadriceps muscles and raise the lower legs slowly until they are extended. Pause at the top and then lower the legs slowly to the starting position. Perform with a controlled movement. Do not kick or swing the legs up. Do not allow the momentum of the weight to move the legs. Exhale on lifting the legs, and inhale on lowering the legs.

Seated Hamstring Curls

Weight Machine.
Targeted area: biceps femoris (long and short head) and gastronemius

Sit on the bench with the legs extended and the back of the ankle on the pads. Contract the torso muscles and slowly pull the lower legs down towards the floor. Pause and then return the legs to the start position.

CORE STRENGTH

A strong core is essential for success in boxing, weight training, and running. Six basic abdominal exercises with suggested repetitions are below. Combine two or three of these exercises together, and perform them at the end of your workout.

Abdominal Crunches

Targeted area: rectus abdominis and oblique abdominis externus

Lie on your back, placing your hands beside the head to give your neck support. Both feet should be placed on the floor with the knees bent. Contract the abdominal muscles, keeping the lower back on the floor. Exhale and lift the head and shoulders up off of the ground as a unit, and move towards the knees. Pause, and then lower the head and shoulders back towards the floor. Repeat, trying to lift the shoulders higher off of the ground. Continue until the muscles feel fatigued or do three sets of thirty repetitions.

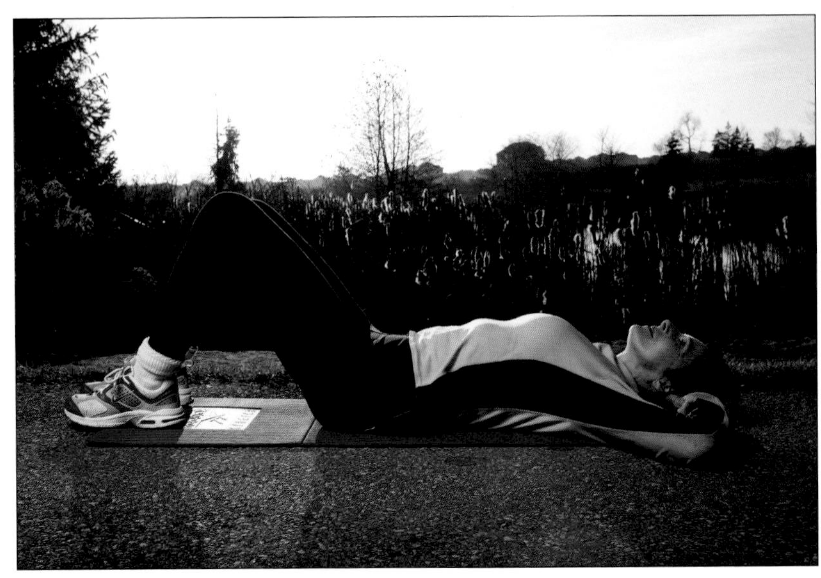

Abdominal crunch–start

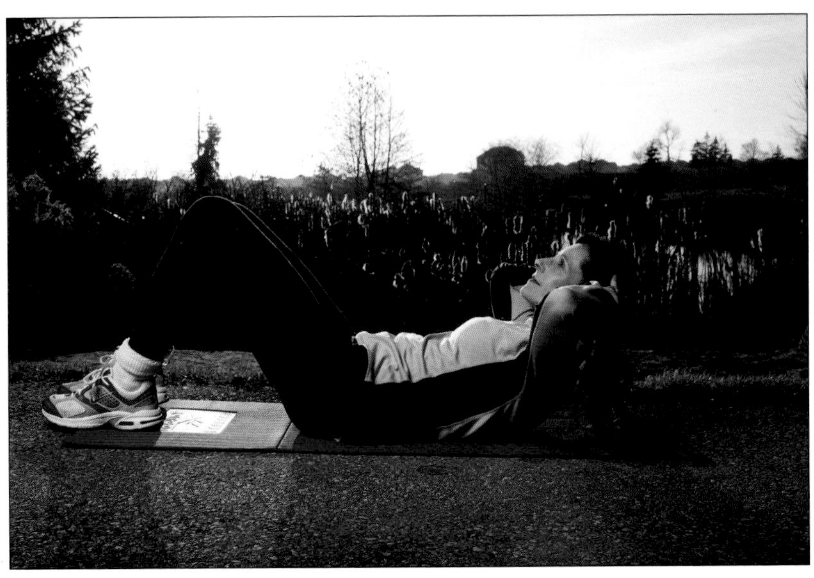

Abdominal crunch–finish

Oblique Crunches

Targeted area: oblique abdominis externus

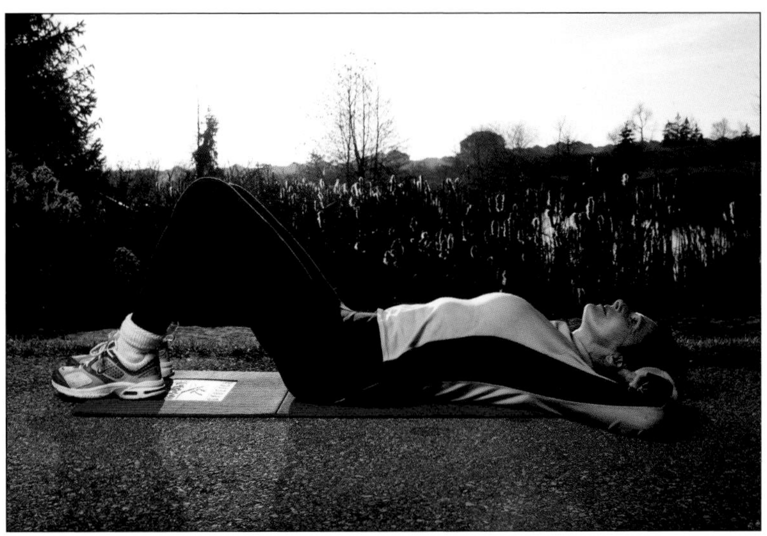

Oblique crunch–start

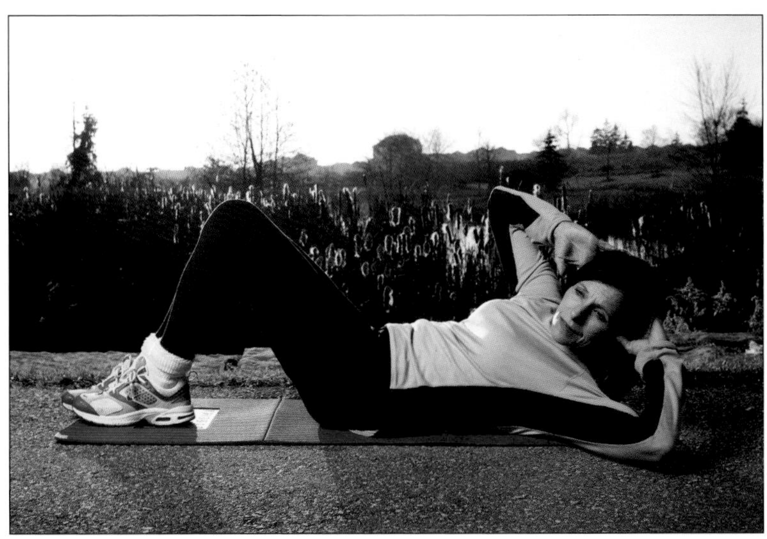

Oblique crunch–finish

Lie on your back as in the abdominal crunches, lift the head and shoulders up off of the floor, and rotate to one side. Come back to the center and lower back to the floor. Repeat to the other side. Repeat until muscles feel fatigued or up to two sets of twenty repetitions. You may also repeat on one side only (fifteen to twenty reps), and repeat on the other side.

Abdominal Leg Press

Targeted area: abdominus externus, tensor fascia lata, rectus femoris, and rectus abdominis

Place your hands on the ground behind your back with elbows slightly bent . Slowly press both legs out, and pull them back in. Lean back slightly as you press your legs forward. For a more difficult version, hold the hands in a boxing position and press the legs out. Try three sets of fifteen reps, with a short rest in between each set.

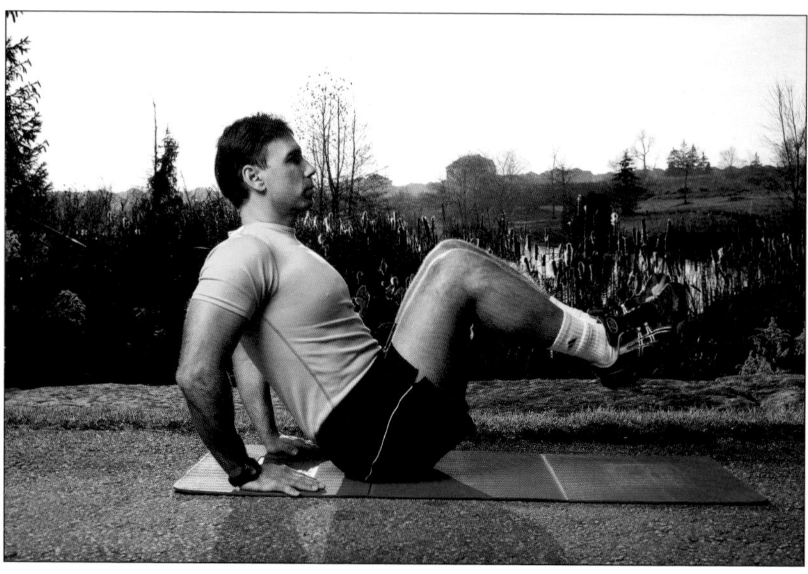

Abdominal leg press–start

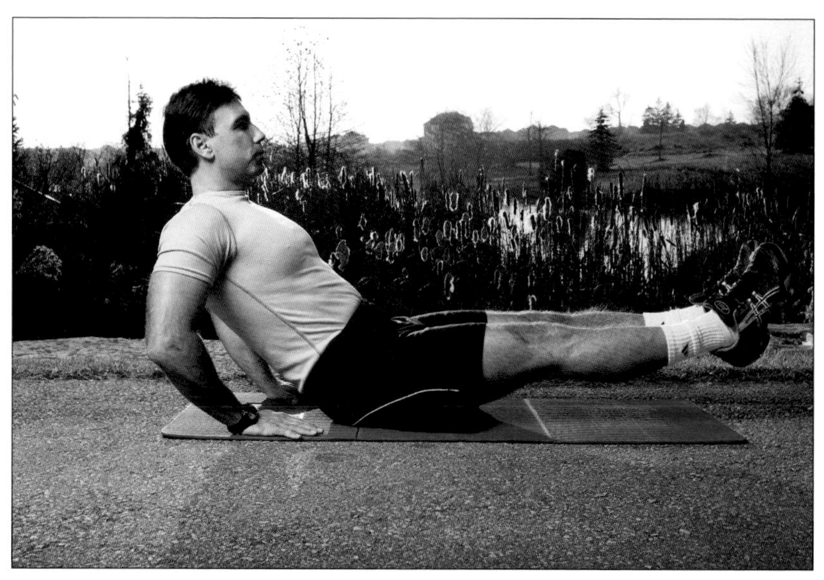

Abdominal leg press–finish

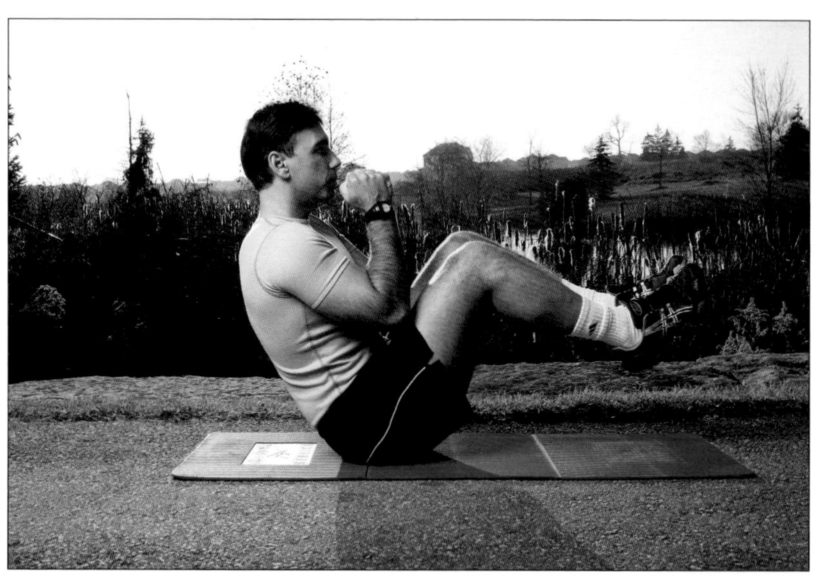

Abdominal leg press (advanced)–start

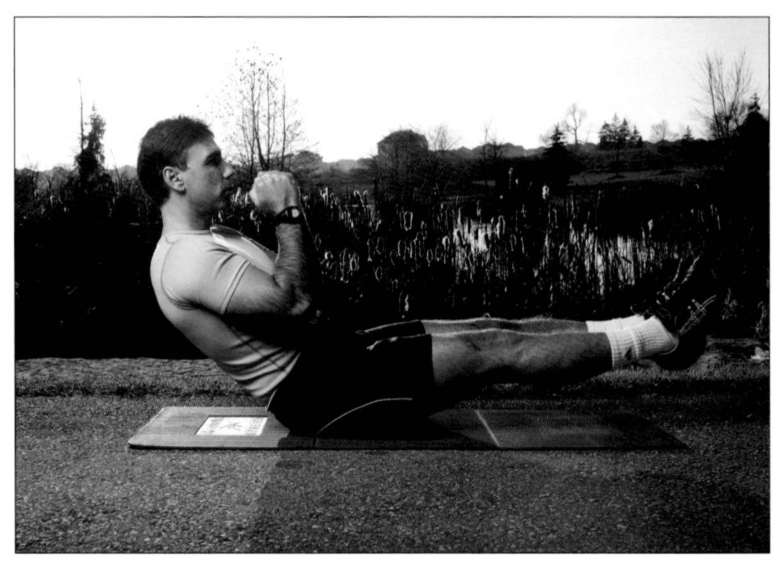

Abdominal leg press (advance)–finish

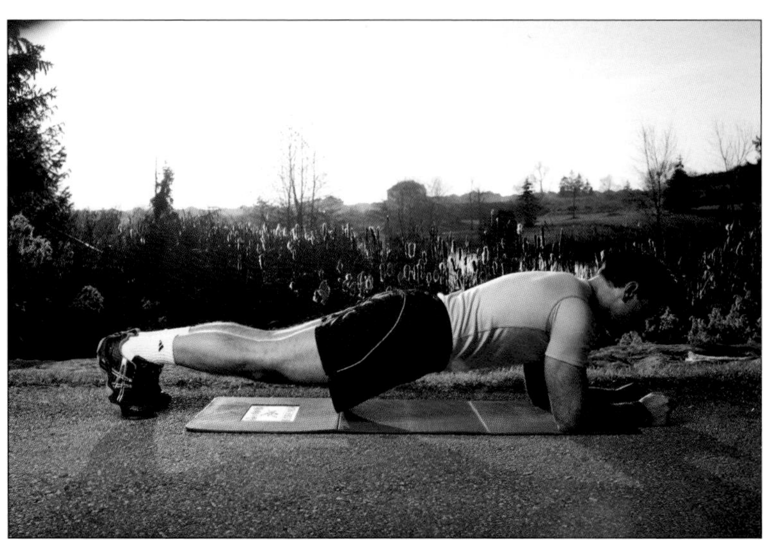

Body plank

Body Plank

Targeted area: rectus abdominis, oblique abdominis externus, and serratus anterior

Position your body with the weight on your elbows and toes, head in line with your back and the body flat. Pull your abs up towards the spine and hold. Try to perform three sets, holding each set for thirty seconds, eventually working up to sixty seconds.

Supine Cycle

Targeted area: abdominis externus, rectus abdominis, oblique abdominis, and rectus femoris

Lie on your back, hands supporting the head and neck, knees in the air, and feet off of the floor. Lift the right shoulder and left knee together, bringing the right elbow close to the left knee. At the same time, extend the right leg at about 45-degrees from the floor. Repeat, bringing the left shoulder and the right knee in (elbow meeting knee) and extending the left leg. Keep the motion continuous, like pedaling a bicycle.

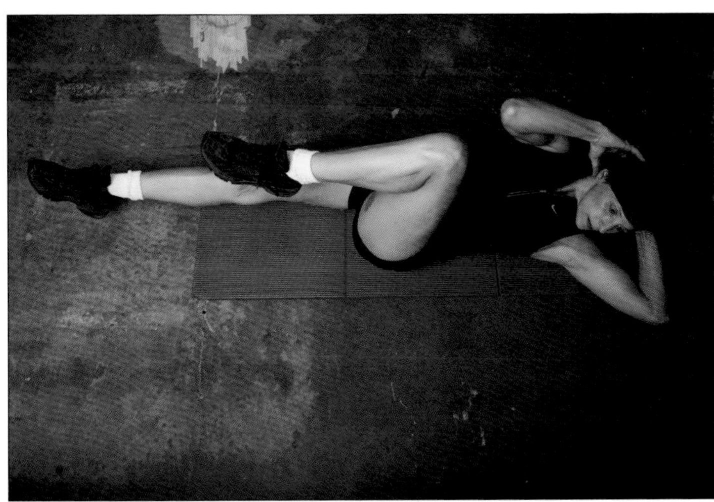

Supine cycle–start

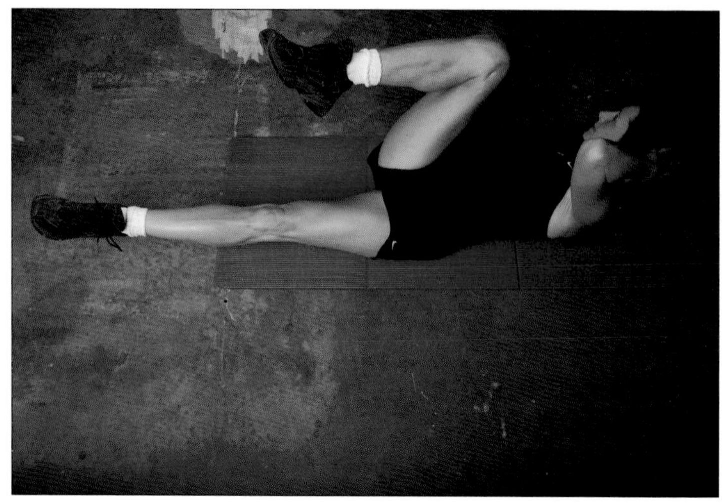

Supine cycle–finish

Back Extension

Targeted area: gluteus maximus and erector spinae

Lie face down, extend the legs, and extend the arms overhead. Keep the torso on the floor. Hold the head held in a straight line with the spine, and lift

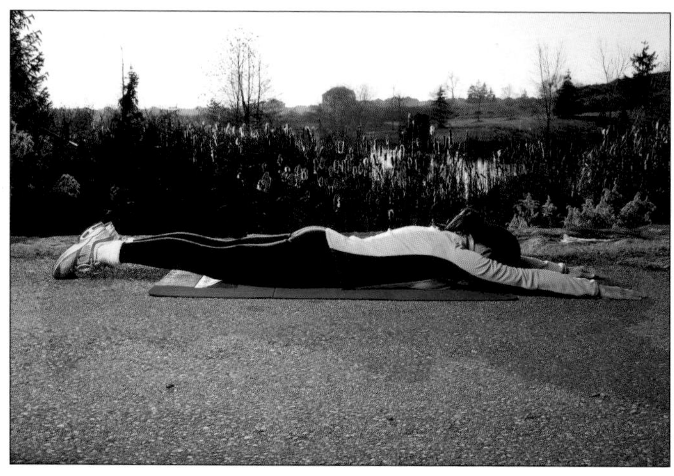

Back extension–start

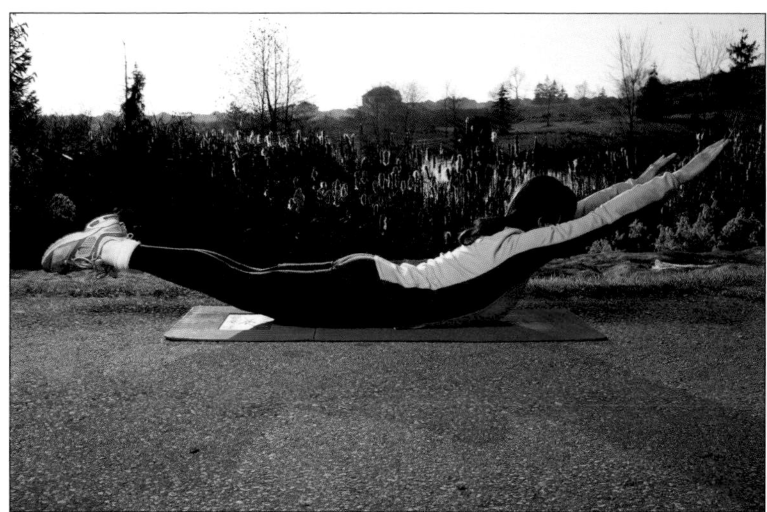

Back extension–finish

both legs and arms off of the floor a few inches. Hold a few seconds, pause, and lower the legs and arms to the floor. You may also lift one leg a time. Repeat until the muscles feel fatigued, or up to fifteen to twenty slow repetitions.

The Medicine Ball

From a boxer's point of view, the medicine ball was designed to condition the abdominal muscles to absorb punishment. The best boxers know that their abdominals must be well armored against attack. The old-time boxing trainer's simple principle states that "the best way to prepare yourself is to absorb blows to the stomach is to absorb blows to the stomach." In preparation for a bout, boxers throw the medicine ball to the abdominal region of a partner, varying the intensity of the throws to simualate a body attack. There are a variety of movements and exercises that use the medicine ball to strengthen the body core and abdominals without making direct contact with the torso. Ranging from two to thirty pounds, the medicine ball can offer a unique and effective workout, not only for the abdominal muscles but also for the back, legs, shoulders, and arms. It allows for a greater range of motion when training

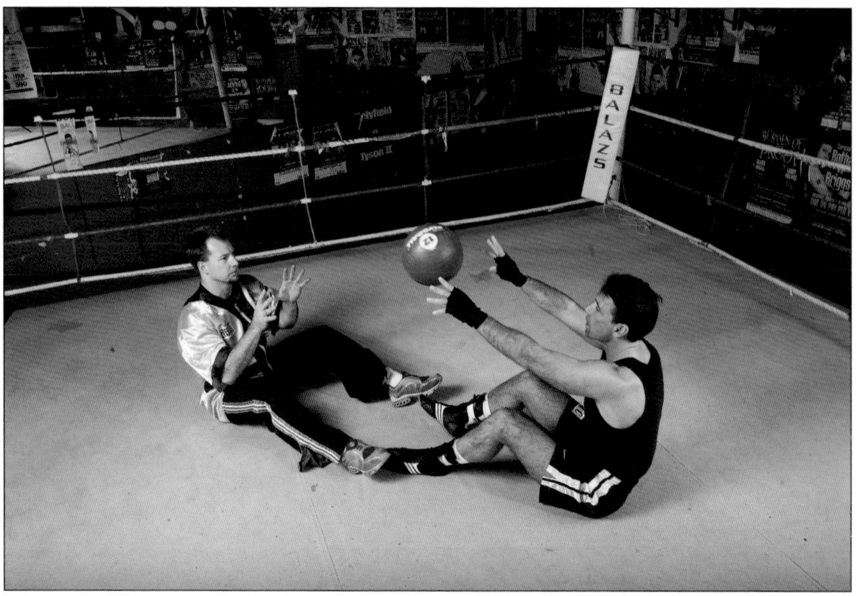

the body core, as compared to weight machines, which can be restrictive and to free weights, which are not conducive to partner-exchange movements.

The greatest advantage of using the medicine ball is that it trains the body core very effectively. It is often difficult to find exercises and training techniques that specifically challenge the main body, but with the use of the medicine ball, all of the torso's musculature is trained to respond to an overload simultaneously. The abdominal muscles and the back muscles are the two major areas of development. The muscles of the arms, chest, and legs can also be strengthened. NOTE: The use of a medicine ball for abdominal strengthening should not even be considered until you feel comfortable performing a series of abdominal crunches and oblique exercises.

Medicine balls have gone through many changes over the years. Traditionally made of black leather, they can now be found in various textures and filled with any number of different materials. We like how Dr. Donald Chu's "Plyoball" medicine ball performs. It is comfortable to hold, has no slip ridges (great for partner-passing drills) and comes in a variety of sizes and weights. Select or combine a few of the medicine balls exercises.

Exercises with the Medicine Ball

Basic Curl-up

Targeted area: rectus abdominis, oblique abdominis externus, quadriceps rectus femoris, and tensor fascia lata

Lie on your back with knees bent and both feet on the floor. Hold the medicine ball on your chest. Control your upper body and head as one unit, and raise them off of the floor until the ball touches your thigh. Return slowly to the floor. Repeat ten to twenty times, one to three sets, with a five- to twelve-pound ball.

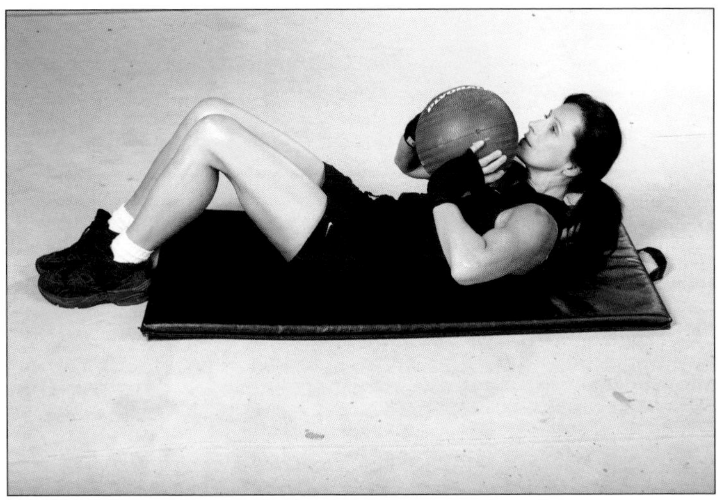

Basic curl-up

Pullover Sit-Up

Targeted area: rectus abdominis, oblique abdominis externus, teres minor, teres major, and deltoids

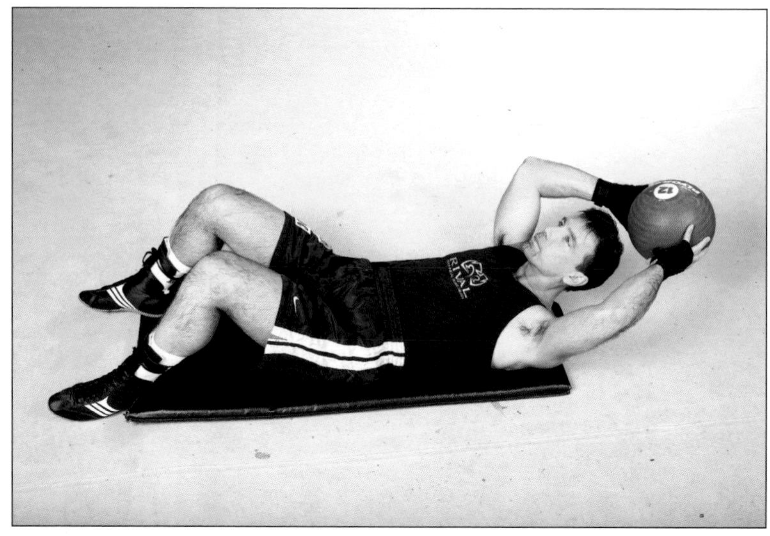

Pullover sit-up–start

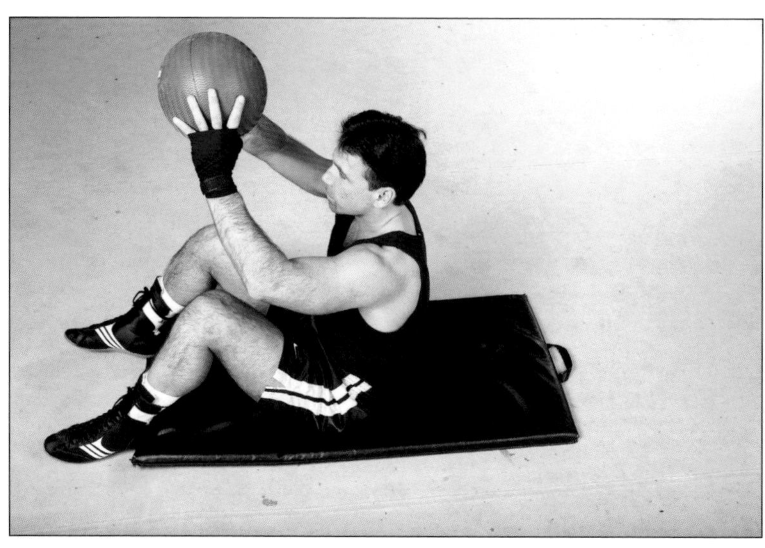

Pullover sit-up–finish

Lie on your back with knees bent and both feet on the floor. Start with the arms fully extended on the floor overhead holding the ball. Bring the ball up overhead and forward towards the chest, and lift the upper body, head, and shoulders off of the floor at about 45 degrees. Return to the starting position, lowering the head and the ball to the floor at the same time. Repeat ten to fifteen times, one to three sets, five- to ten-pound ball.

Hip Crunch

Targeted area: rectus abdominis, oblique abdominis externus, rectus femoris, and tensor fascia lata

Sit with knees bent and feet on the floor. Extend the arms behind the body and place the hands on the floor for support. Squeeze the ball between the knees. Raise the feet off of the floor and pull the knees and ball towards the chest. Return the knees and feet to the starting position. Repeat ten to fifteen times, one to three sets, with a five- to ten-pound ball.

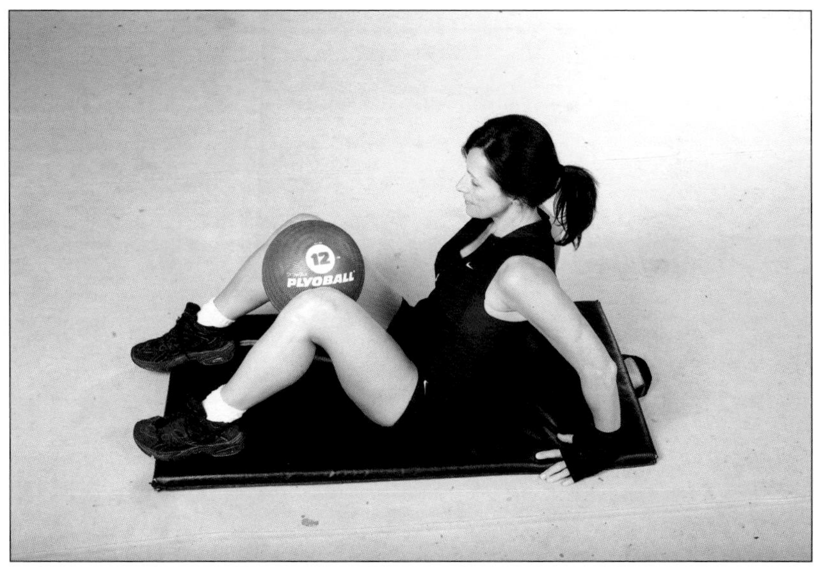

Hip crunch–start

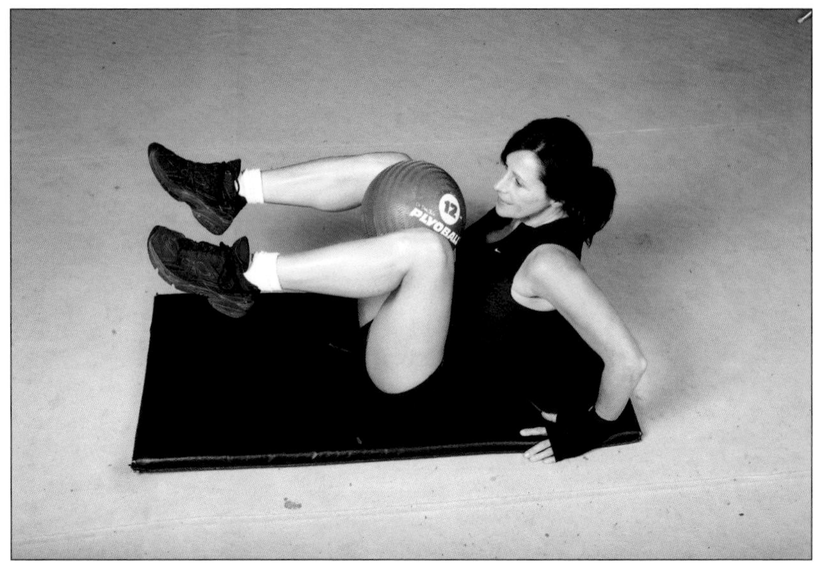

Hip crunch–finish

Oblique Twist

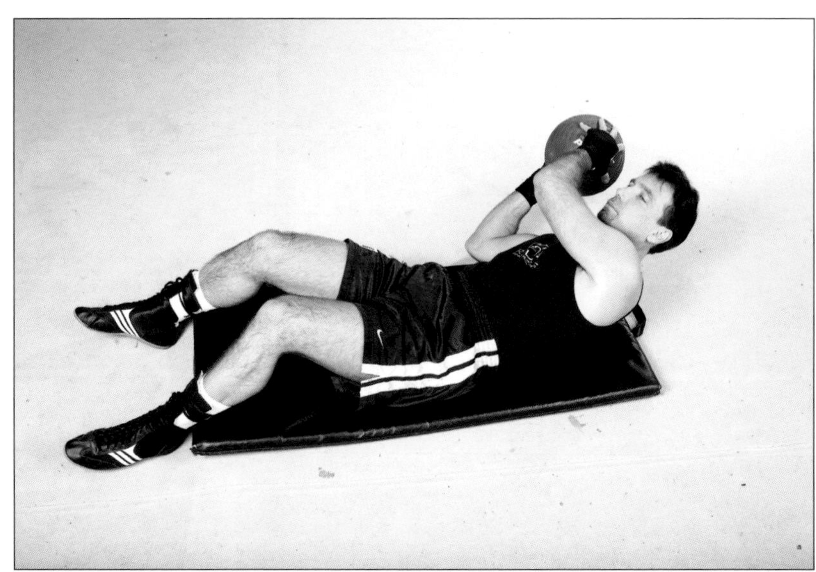

Oblique twist–start

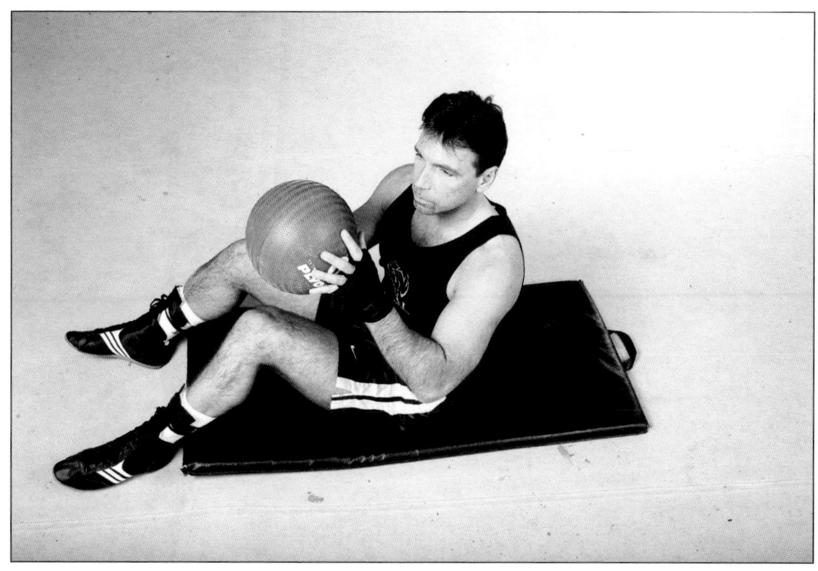

Oblique twist–finish

Targeted area: rectus abdominis, and oblique abdominis externus

Lie on your back with knees bent and both feet on the floor. Hold the medicine ball over the right shoulder area with both hands. Simultaneously lift the upper body and the ball up towards the right knee. Lower your back slowly to the start position. Continue on one side for the full number of repetitions, and then repeat on the other side. Repeat ten to fifteen times, one to two sets, with a five- to ten-pound ball.

Hip Raises

Targeted area: rectus abdominis, tensor fascia lata, quadriceps rectus femoris, oblique abdominus externus, gracilis, and adductors

Lie on your back with your hands beside your head, legs extended straight over the hips, and the ball squeezed between the legs. Hold this position and lift the hips up. Then lower back to the floor slowly and with control. Repeat ten to fifteen times, one to three sets, with a three- to five-pound ball.

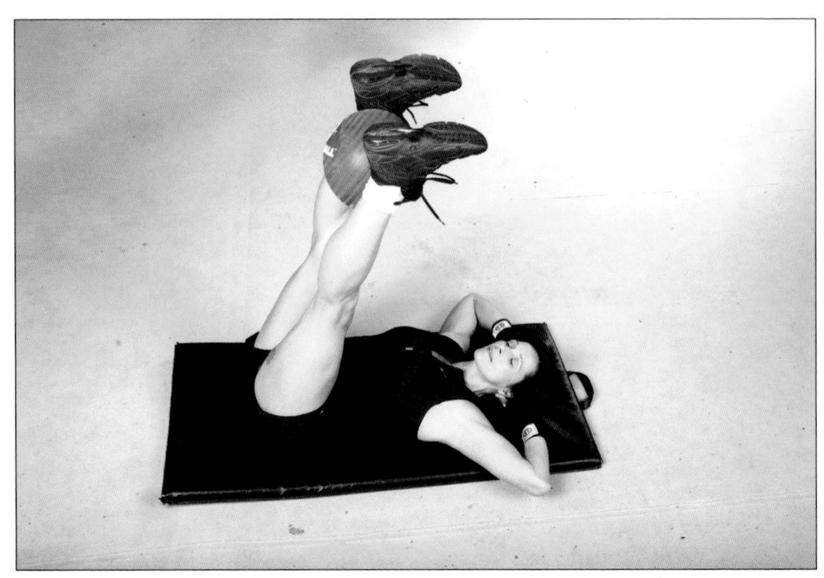

Hip raise–start

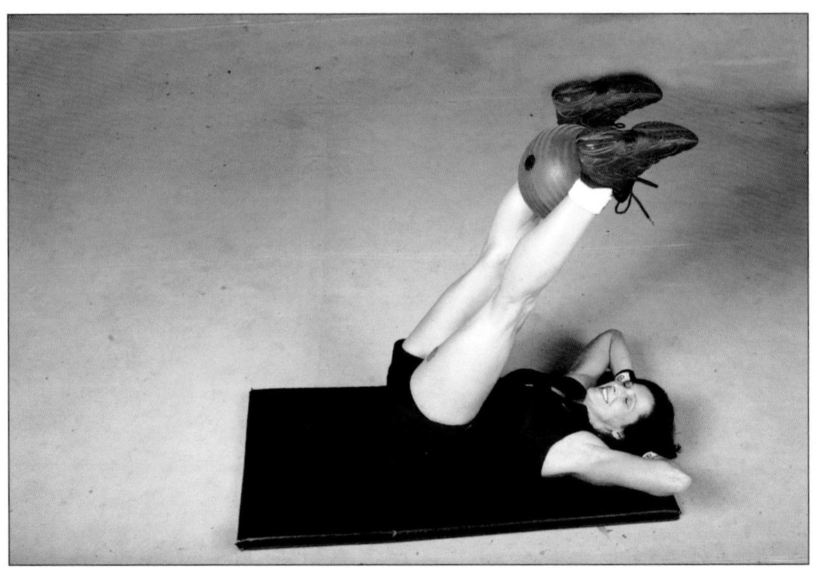

Hip raise–finish

Single Leg V-Ups

Targeted area: rectus abdominis, tensor fascia lata, and quadriceps rectus femoris

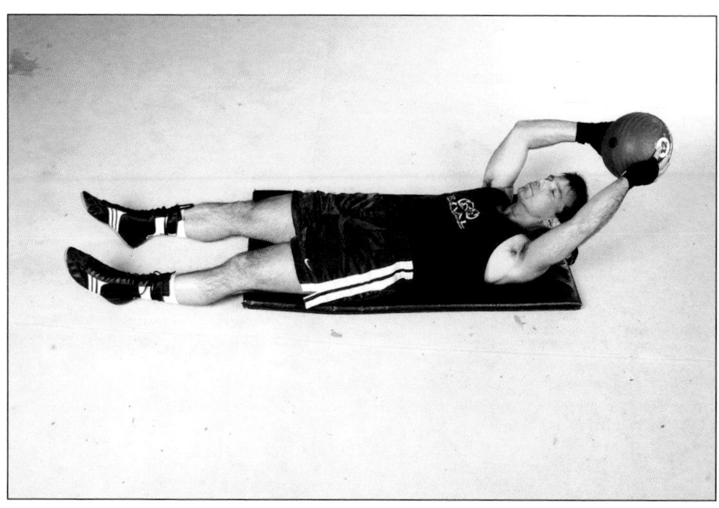

Single Leg V-ups–start

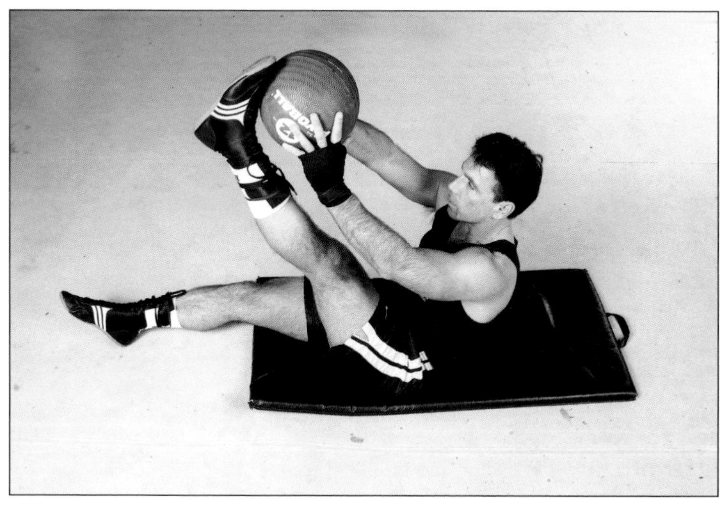

Single Leg V-ups–finish

Lie back onto floor with the knees bent. The head should be in a neutral position, with a space between the chin and chest. Hold the ball over your head with arms extended while raising the trunk 45 degrees. At the same time, lift one leg to meet the ball and return to the start position. Repeat lifting the other leg. This is a great exercise, which will develop strength in the lower portion of the abdominal muscles and the hip flexors.

Double V-Ups (Advanced)

Targeted area: rectus abdominis, tensor fascia lata, and quadriceps rectus femoris

Lying on your back with the legs extended and the medicine ball held overhead, contract the abdominal muscles and raise the arms, body, and both legs simultaneously in a smooth motion, attaining a V-position. Return to the lying position by lowering the legs and body together in a controlled manner. Always maintain proper body alignment, leg extension, and arm position.

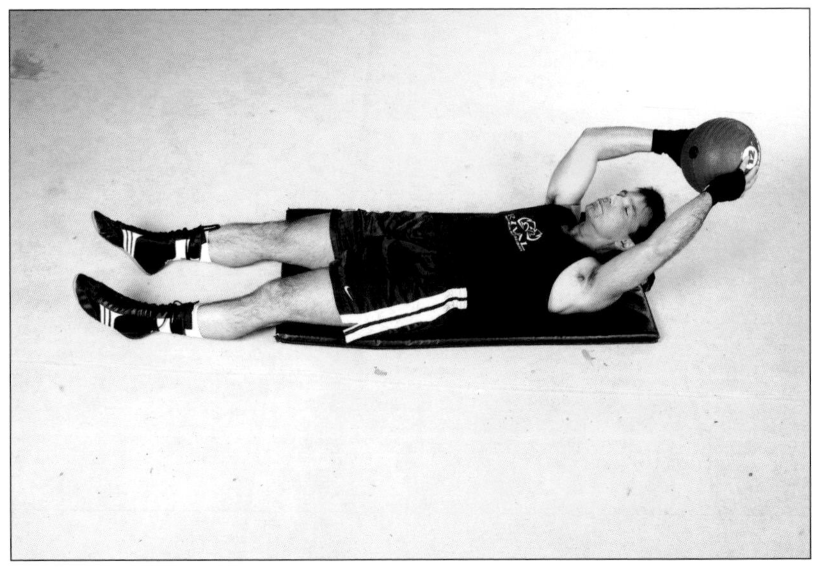

Double V-ups–start

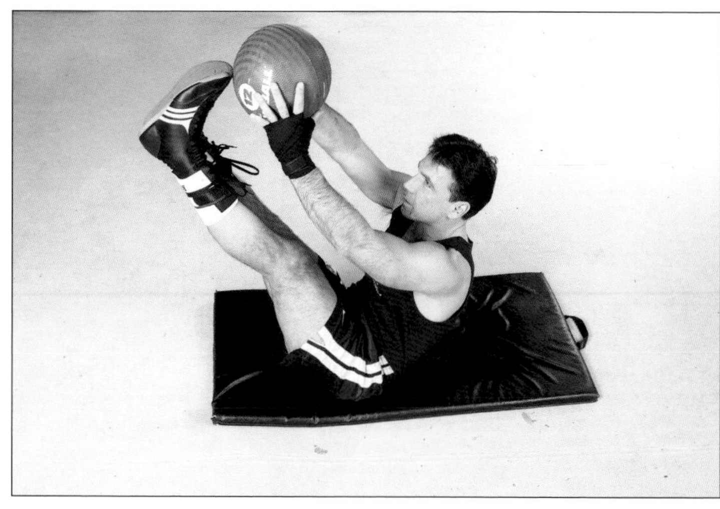

Double V-ups–finish

Partner Twist

Targeted area: oblique abdominus externus, oblique abdominus internus, and latissimus dorsi.

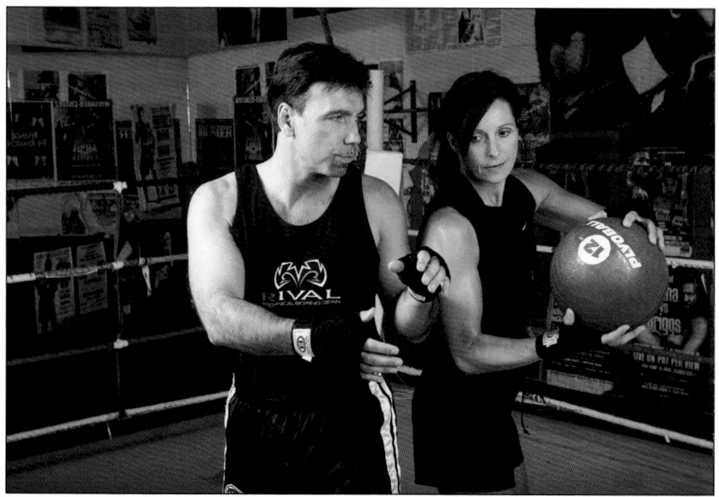

Partner twist–twist to one side

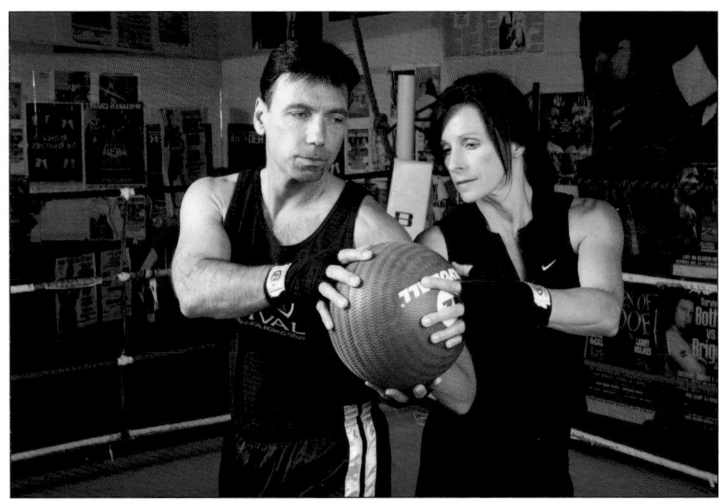

Partner twist–hand the ball off

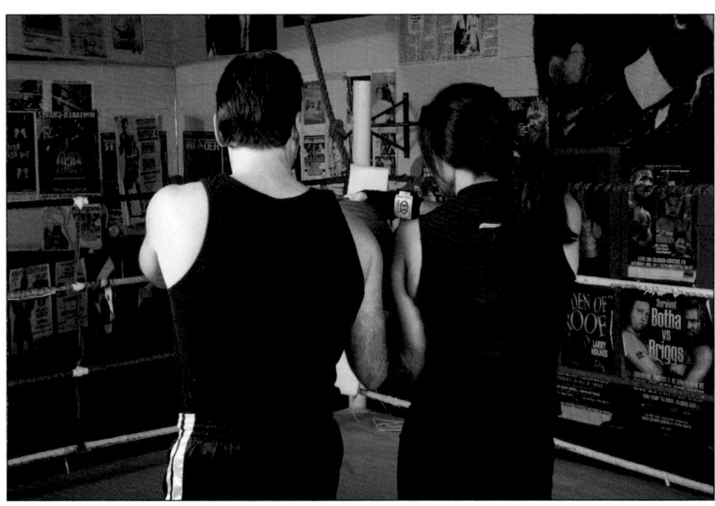

Partner twist–twist to the other side

Stand back-to-back with a partner. Rotate the body and pass the ball to your partner. To increase difficulty, increase the distance between you and your partner. Repeat ten to fifteen times, one to three sets, with a five- to ten-pound ball.

Sit-up Toss

Targeted area: rectus abdominis, oblique abdominis externus, teres minor, teres major, and deltoids

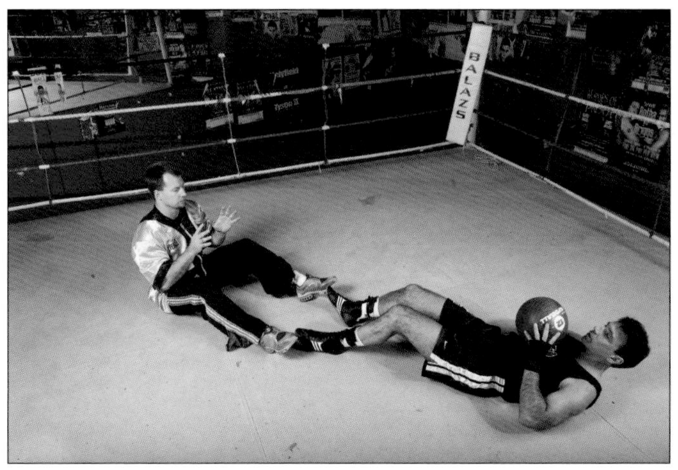

Sit-up toss–sit ready to catch the ball

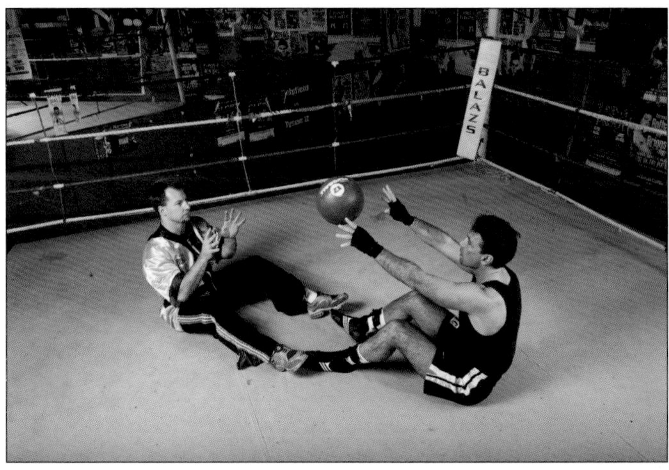

Sit-up toss–toss the ball

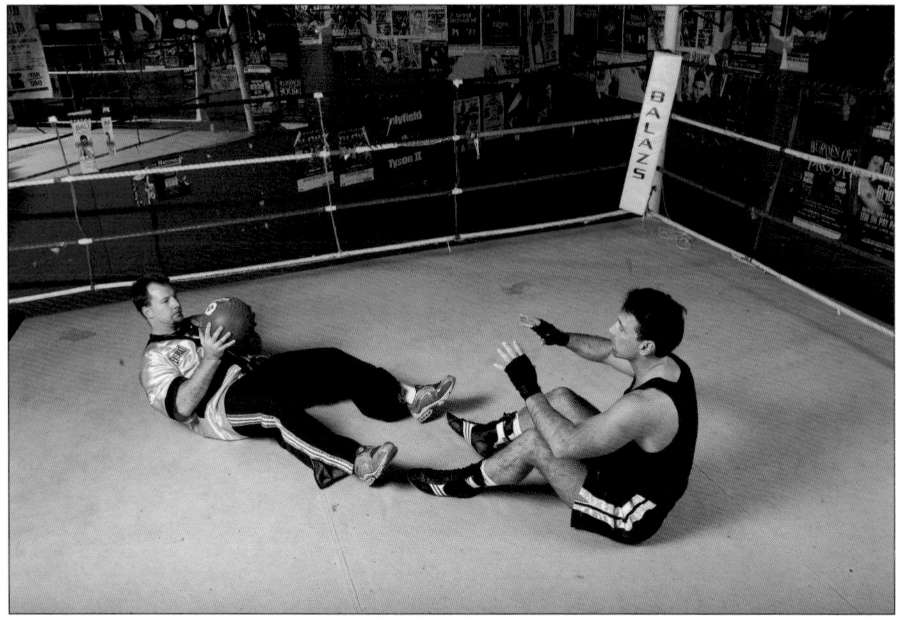

Sit-up toss–catch the ball

Sit on the floor with knees bent and arms in front of you ready to catch a ball toss. Your partner sits approximately three to four feet away. As you catch the ball, slowly lower your trunk to the floor in a controlled manner. Sit back up, tossing the ball to your partner. Repeat, remembering to keep your feet on the floor, eyes on your partner, and shoulders square over the hips.

Lower Body Muscles

Overhead Squats

Targeted area: gluteus maximus, gluteus medius, quadriceps, and deltoids

Stand with the feet shoulder-width apart, and hold the ball at waist level. As you lower into a squat position, raise the medicine ball overhead. Keep the center of gravity over the heels, back straight, and head in line with the spine. Hold the squat position for two counts, and return to the start. Repeat ten to fifteen times, one to three sets, with a ten- to twenty-five-pound ball.

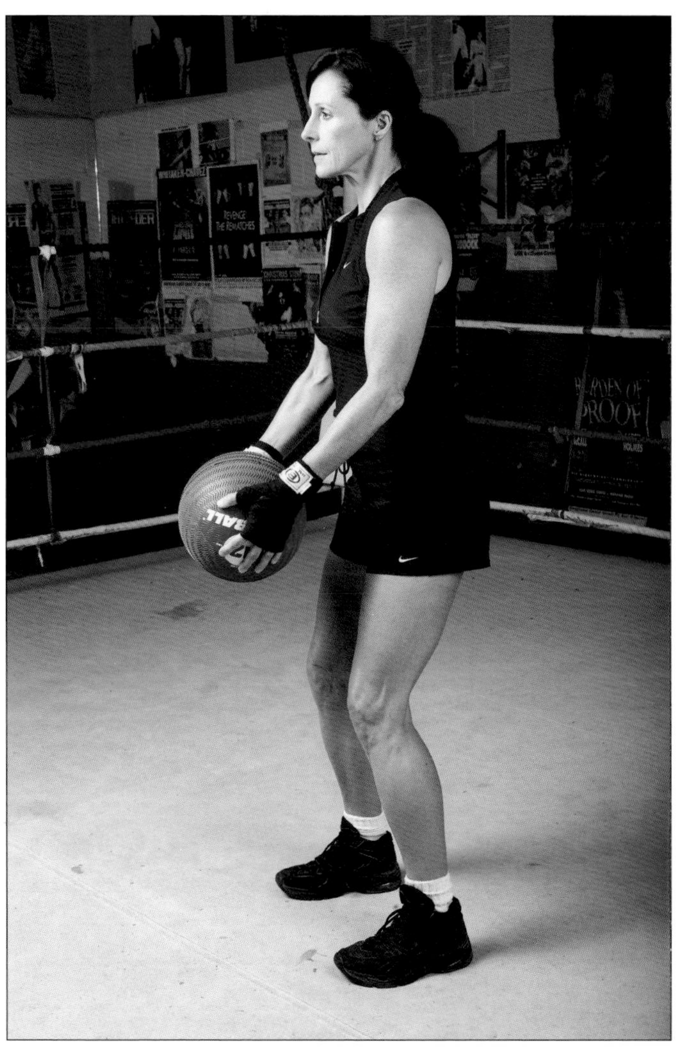

Overhead squat–start

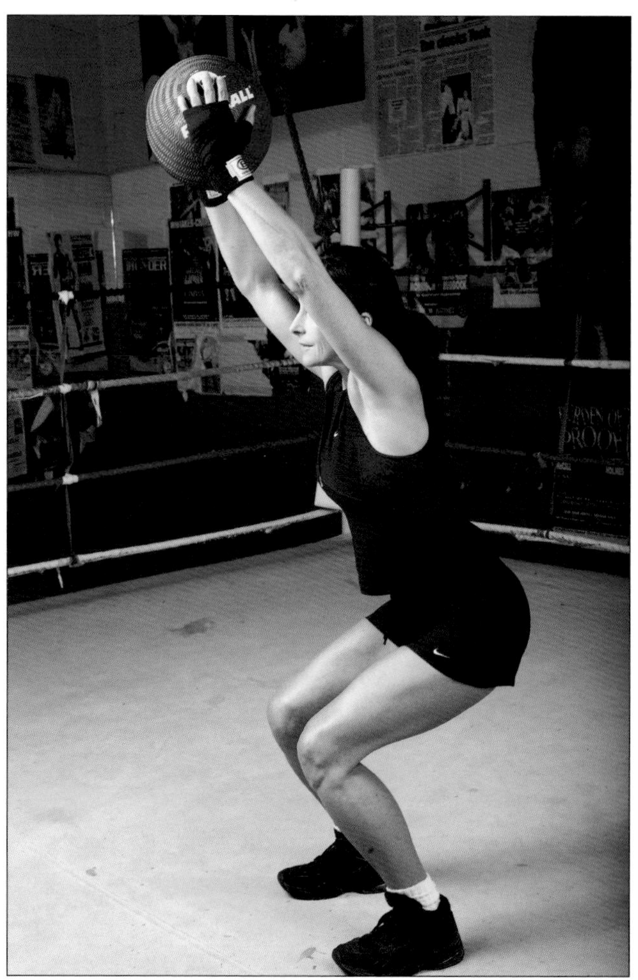

Overhead squat–finish

Power Squats (Advanced)

Targeted area: gluteus maximus, gluteus medius, quadriceps, soleus, gastroncnemius, and plantaris

Stand with the feet shoulder-width apart, and hold the ball in front of you close to the chest. As you lower into a squat position, keep the center of gravity

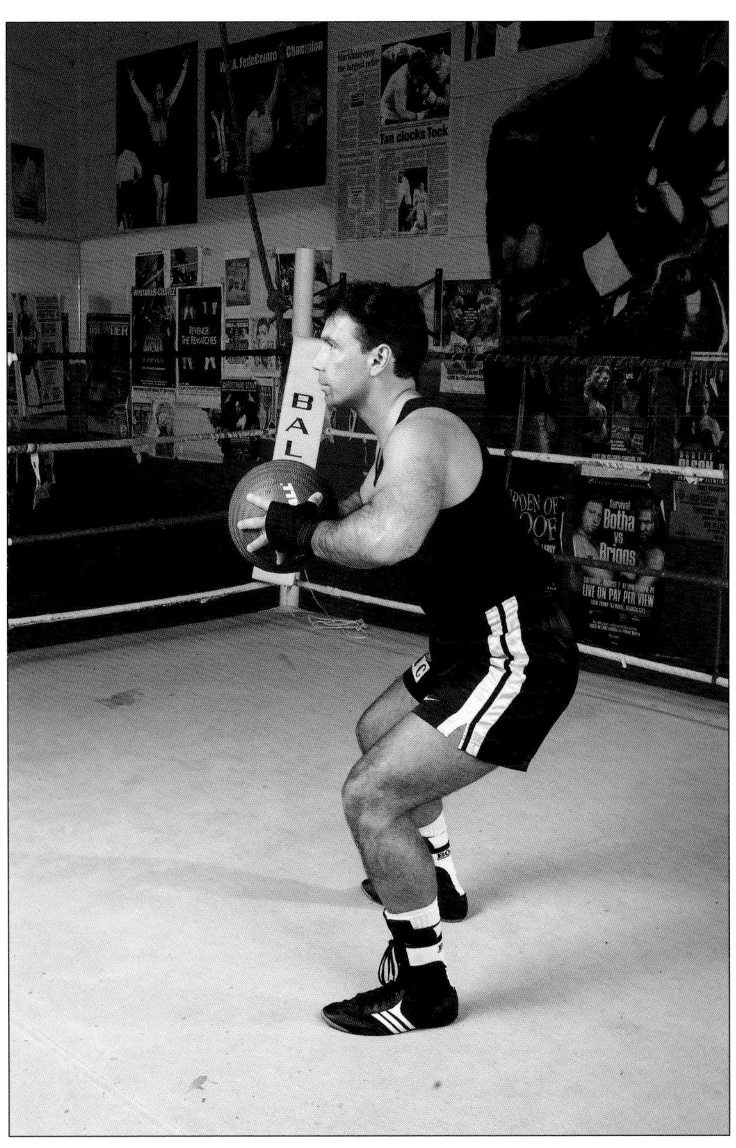

Power squat–start

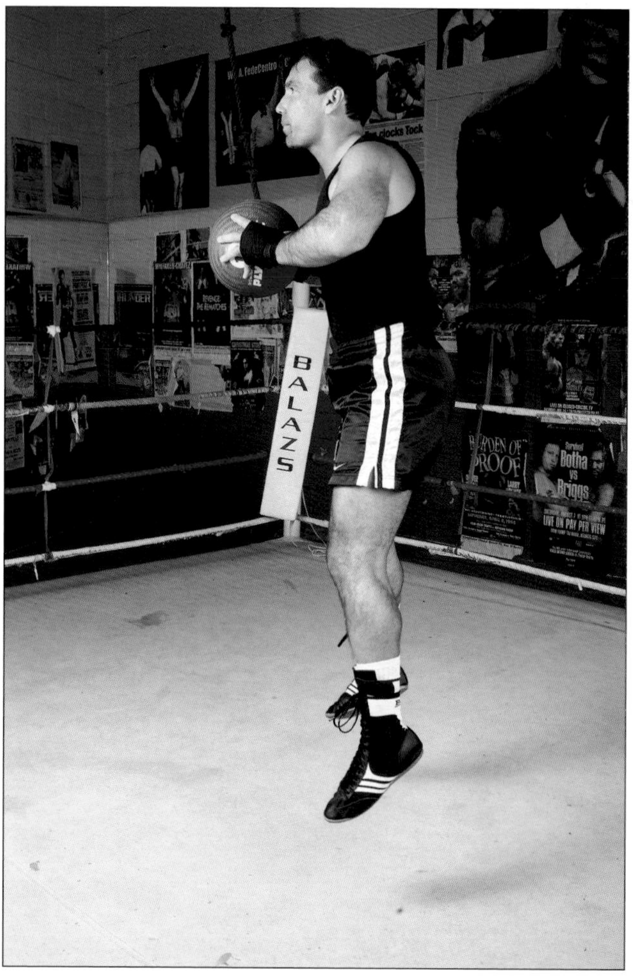

Power squat–finish

over the heels, back straight, and head in line with the spine. Pause and then explode upward, extending the legs and pushing off with the feet. Land on the floor in a controlled manner, rolling through the balls of the feet and attaining the squat position. Pause and then jump again. Repeat ten to fifteen times, one to two sets, with a ten- to twenty-five-pound ball.

Forward Lunges

Targeted area: gluteus maximus, quadriceps, and biceps femoris (long and short head)

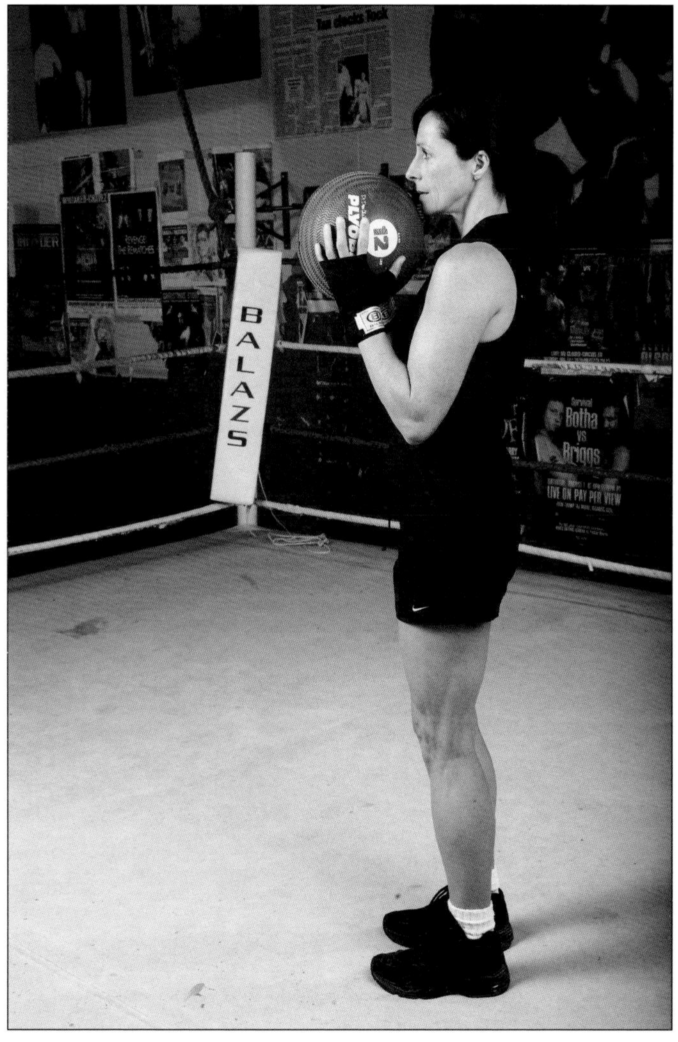

Forward lunge–start

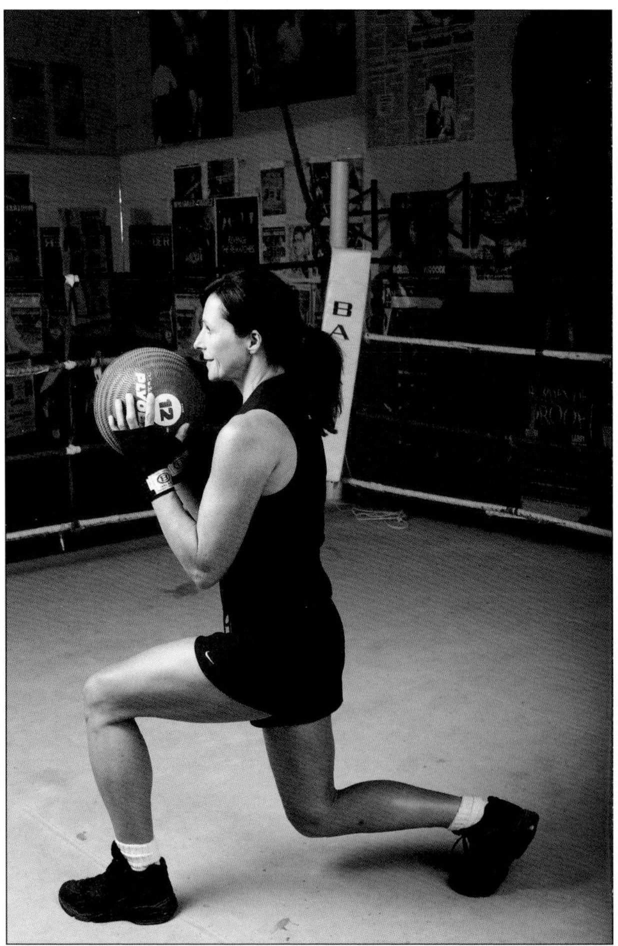

Forward lunge–finish

Stand with the ball held at chest level and the feet shoulder-width apart. Step forward, and lower your body onto the forward leg. Push back off your front foot to return to your starting position, and repeat. When stretched fully, your upper body should be perpendicular to your front thigh, and your back knee should be lower than your front knee. Don't let your front knee bend past 90 degrees. Switch legs and repeat.

Upper Body Muscles

Off-Set Push-ups (Advanced)

Targeted area: pectoralis major, and serratus anterior

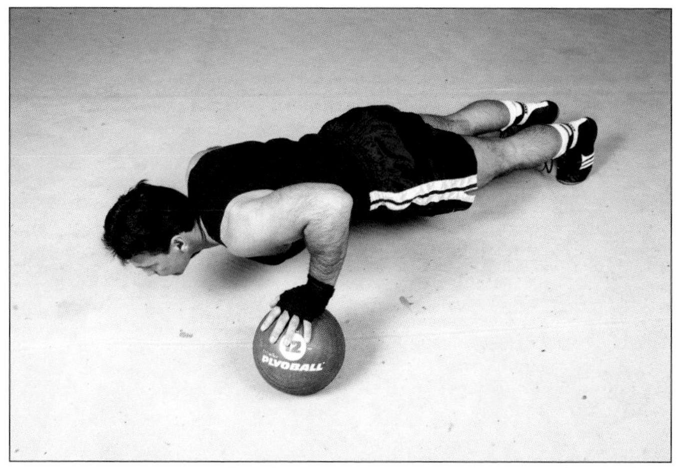

Off-set push-up–start

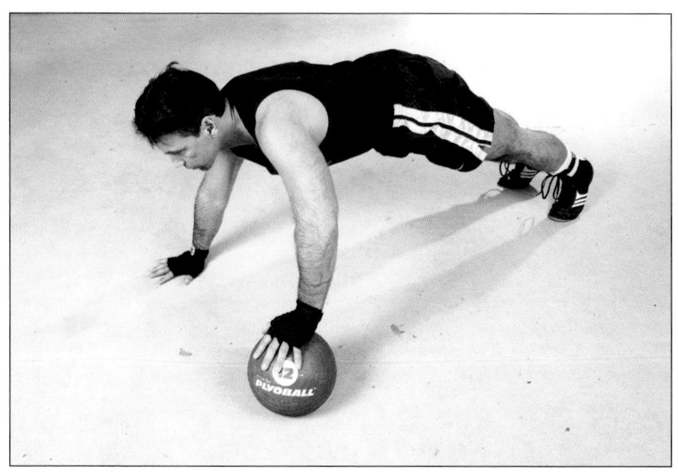

Off-set push-up–finish

In the push-up position, put the ball under one hand. The ball represents somewhat of an unstable surface, which makes these pushups much more difficult than regular pushups. This forces the stabilizers of the shoulder and rotator cuff muscles to work very hard to keep the shoulder joint steady while performing the exercise. Switch the ball to the other hand and repeat. Make sure you perform these push-ups in a slow controlled motion and exhale on the exertion as you're pushing up.

The Boxer's Push-Up (Advanced)

Targeted area: pectoralis major, and serratus anterior

Start with both hands on the medicine ball and the body in a push-up position. Lower the body towards the ground keeping the elbows pointing back and the abdominals held tight. The hands are held close together and must be kept steady. These push-ups require additional strength through the torso, arms, and shoulders to maintain a perfect balance.

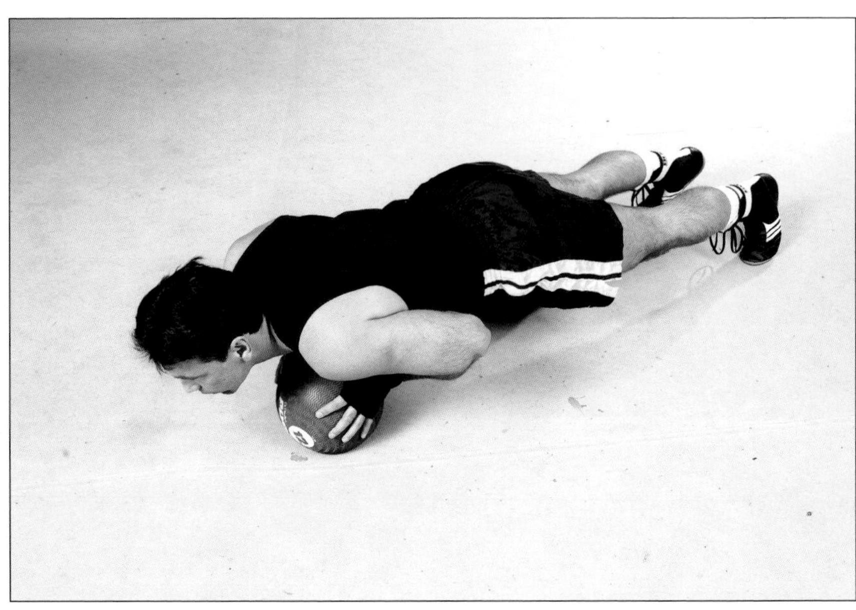

Boxer's push-up–start

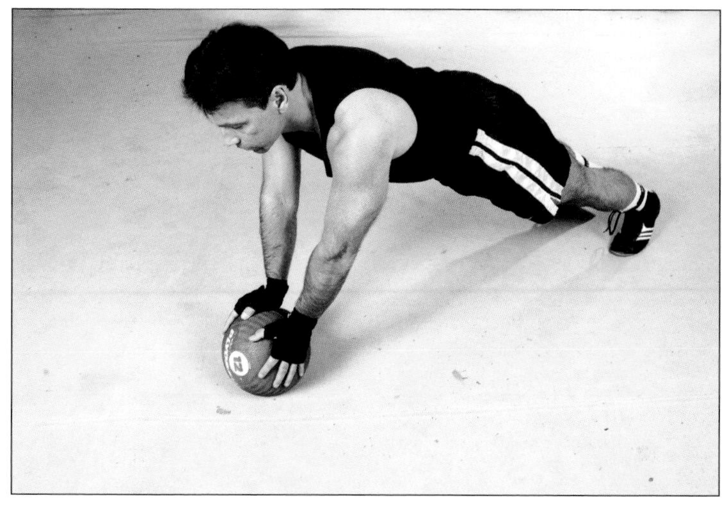

Boxer's push-up–finish

Kneel to Push-Ups (Advanced)

Targeted area: pectoralis major, and serratus anterior

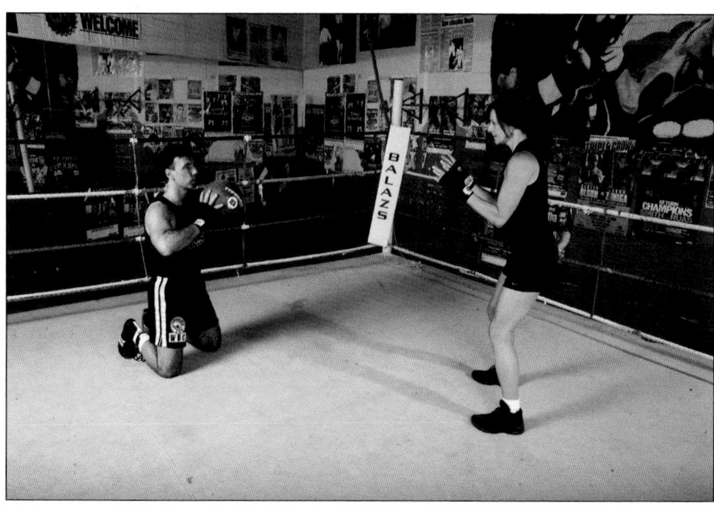

Kneel to push-up–start

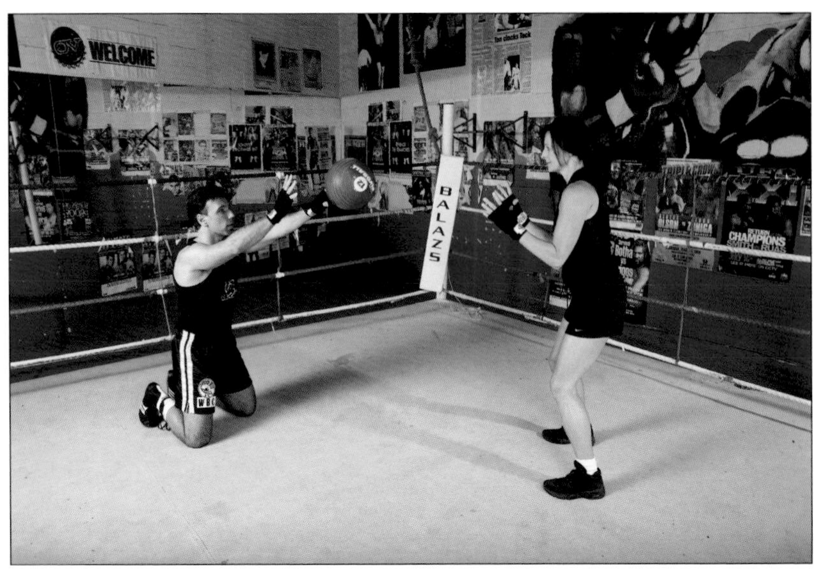

Kneel to push-up–toss the ball

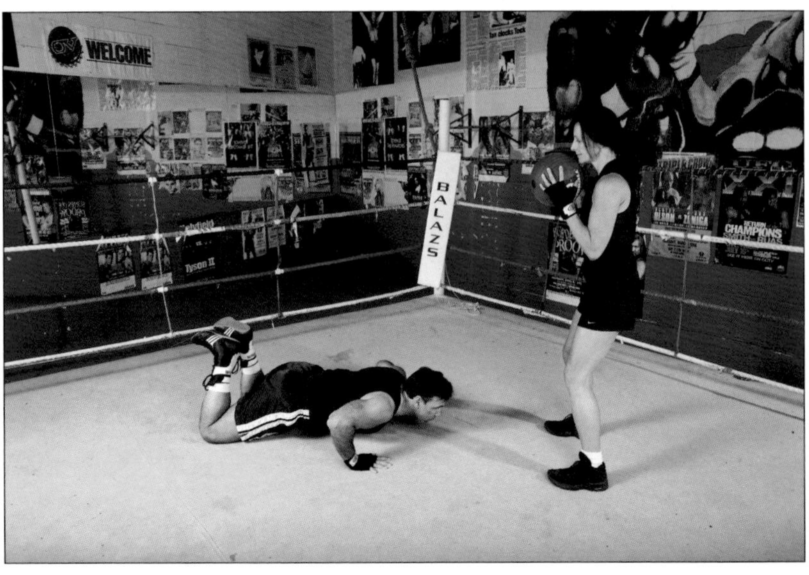

Kneel to push-up–catch the ball/perform a push-up

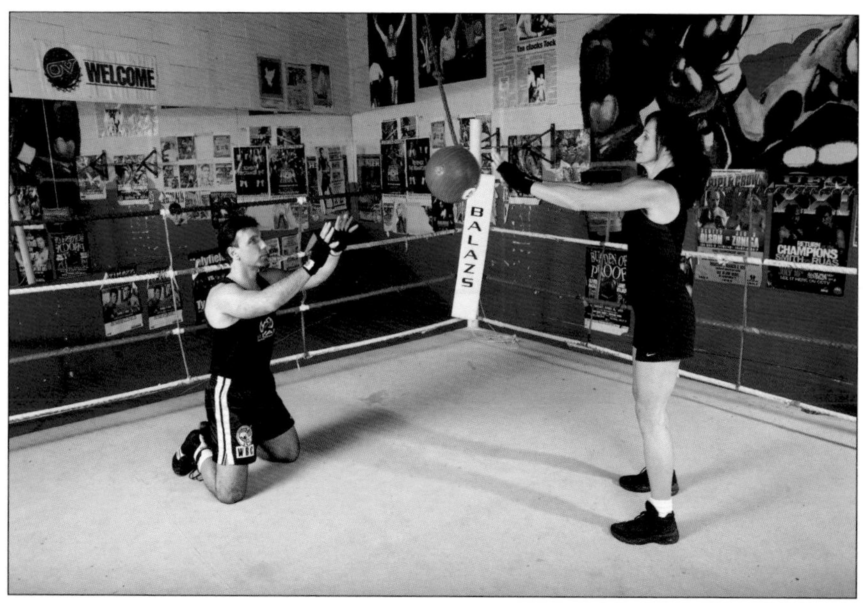

Kneel to push-up–toss the ball back

Your body starts in an upright position sitting on your knees. Hold the medicine ball at chest level. Keeping your torso erect, fall forward as you throw the medicine ball to your partner, using a chest pass. Upon releasing the ball, drop your hands to the floor and immediately complete a push-up. Explode as you complete the push-up to obtain the starting upright position on your knees. Your partner throws the ball back to you. Repeat. Try three sets of six to eight reps.

What's Right About Boxing

10

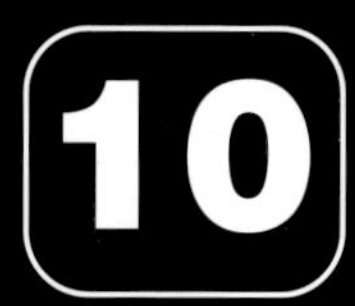

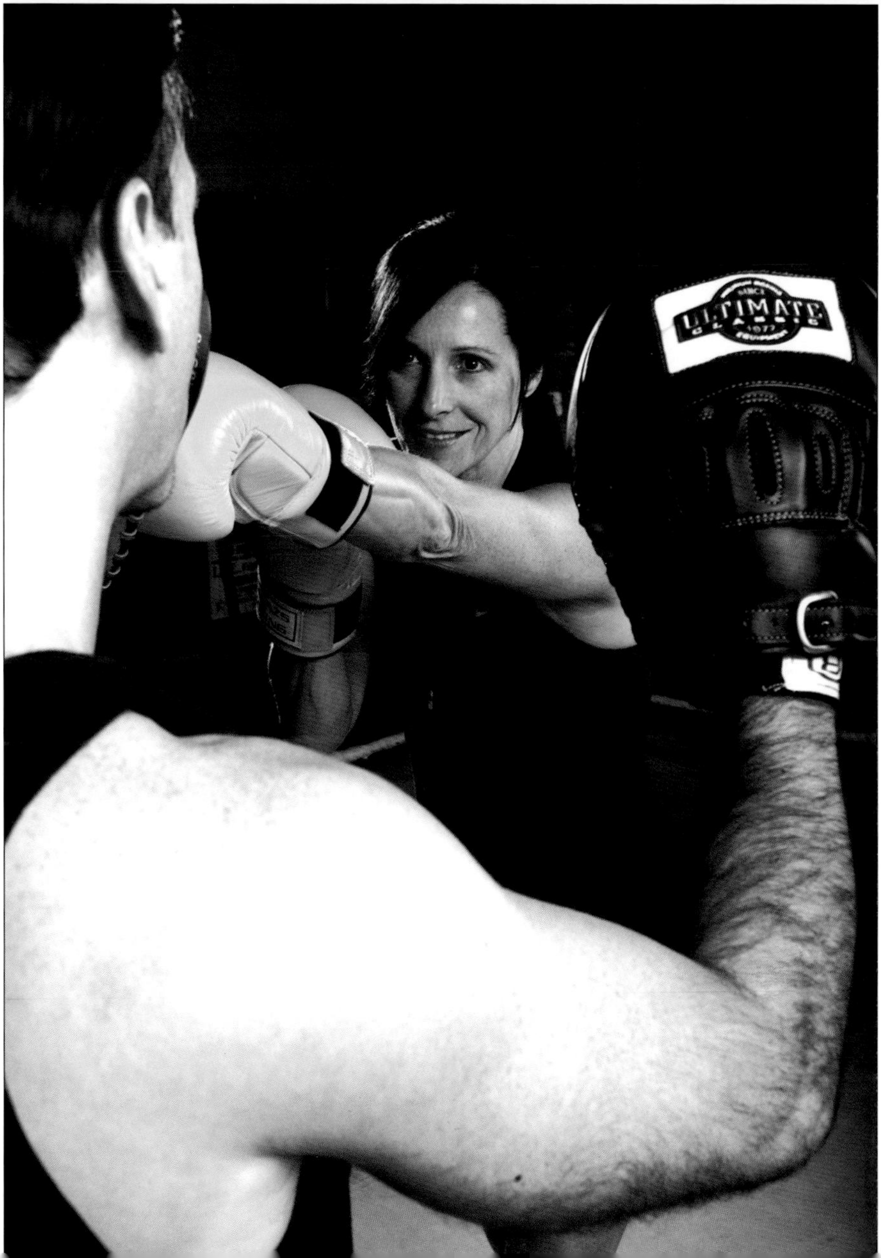

Boxing teaches you to rely on yourself, value the input of others, and respect both your own skills and those of others. It is rewarding and challenging; promotes athleticism, physical and mental conditioning, sportsmanship and self-worth; and is one of the most challenging activities that you will ever do. Boxing is a great vehicle to release tension, stress, and frustrations, and it builds self-confidence and character. Amateur boxing is not about knocking your opponent out. It is about developing a skill, improving your fitness level, and setting goals.

For most, fitness boxing is enough. Hitting the heavy bag, working the speed bag, and jumping rope provide a challenging, creative way to stay fit and release stress. Some, however, may want to take it a step further and participate in controlled sparring. If you are ready for the next challenge, find a serious boxing club, start to work with a trainer, and get prepared to step into the ring.

Looking for a Boxing Club

Walking into a boxing club is seeing, hearing, and experiencing raw energy. And there is really nothing like it. The first thing that will draw your attention is the boxing ring. You'll notice the unique feeling of climbing through the ropes to shadow box and move around, the sound of the speed bag, the rhythmic pounding of the heavy bag, whirling hands and feet, and coaches yelling commands to the fighters. If you were not in the mood to work out before, you quickly get caught up in the atmosphere. Everyone has similar goals, and working hard is contagious.

Every club is different, but there are some basic things to look for. There should be a variety of heavy bags, double-end bags, and speed bags. Look for a conditioning area for both a cardiovascular and a muscle-conditioning workout, large mirrors to check your punching technique, a ring, target mitts, and boxing gloves. There should be changing facilities, times that are convenient for your workout schedule, and water available.

Most clubs offer lessons for small groups, or you may prefer private instruction with a certified trainer or coach. Many fitness clubs now offer a space for good non-contact boxing workouts (no sparring), but serious boxing clubs dedicate space, a ring, equipment, and coaching specific to sparring and contact boxing.

Ensure that the atmosphere and the management are what you are looking for. The boxers training in the club should be dedicated, motivated, and hard working. Club members should include both professionals and amateurs. The owners and the trainers should be approachable and well informed about fitness training, boxing certification, rules, and regulations.

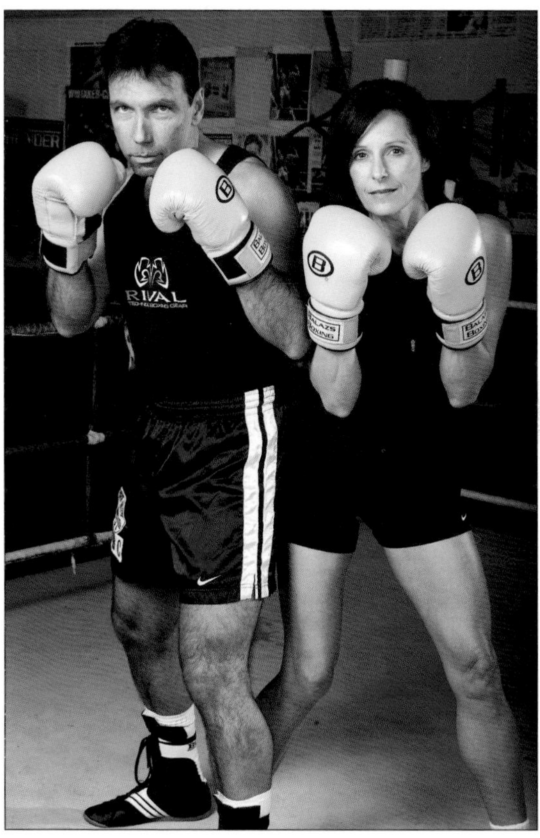

Sparring

Sparring gives you a chance to try out all the moves that you have been practicing while shadow boxing, working on the bags, and it gives you an opportunity to improve all aspects of your game. Sparring allows you to practice offensive punches and introduces the defensive nature of the sport. You have to improvise your next move, and it is more complicated and intense than throwing punches on the heavy bag or with target mitts. Everything that you have practiced now has to be performed under pressure. The purpose of sparring is to fine-tune your skills and simulate fight conditions in a controlled environment.

Sparring is not for everyone. Heavy bags don't hit back; sparring partners do. You should be developing technical and physical skills for a minimum of six months before sparring. If you want to experience it, you have to be in great physical condition. You should be able to go four or five rounds on the heavy bag (at a fast pace), run five to six miles (including sprints), and jump rope for at least fifteen to twenty minutes. Hitting and getting hit takes a lot of getting used to. Sparring should always be taken seriously and recognized as a potentially dangerous activity.

Find a serious boxing club, and only spar under the supervision of an experienced, certified boxing instructor. Protective equipment is necessary, and headgear, a mouthpiece, and a groin protector, and chest protector for females must be worn. Sparring is done in the boxing ring, on a cushioned surface, and not on a hard floor surface. Both boxers wear large sparring gloves (at least sixteen ounces) and listen to and follow the coach's instructions.

Directed Sparring

With directed sparring, each boxer is given a set of instructions on what types of punches to throw. Sessions may include one boxer working on defensive moves (deflecting and slipping punches) and the other working on offensive moves (throwing punches). The trainer may switch roles and will add more elements into the sparring as the training continues. Directed sparring allows the boxer to gain confidence before advancing to free-form sparring.

Situational sparring works on specific drills and helps familiarize the boxer with different fighting styles. The boxer develops muscle memory and quick reflexes. You will then start to develop your own fighting style as you experience sparring in different situations and with different opponents.

As a novice, your trainer should have you work with an experienced boxer, who will not take advantage of your lack of experience and make sure that

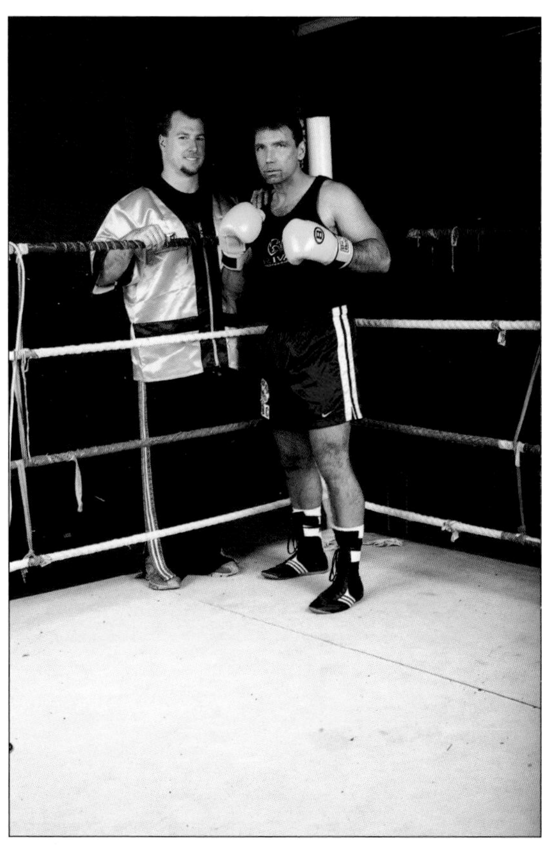

you and your sparring partner agree on the pace and intensity of your sparring workout.

What to Look For in a Trainer

A trainer should be certified with one of the national boxing associations and have experience training a successful boxer, whether an amateur or professional boxer. You want a trainer who knows the game inside out and has a love of the sport.

Ensure that the trainer is approachable and listens to what you want, so that a program can be designed for your needs. The trainer needs to be willing to share his or her successes and training beliefs freely and have enough time to commit to a training session at least once per week. A commitment from you is also necessary to work out in unsupervised sessions, doing roadwork, working the bag, and practicing what the trainer has taught you. Your commitment and the trainer's commitment are important to reach your goals.

Watch a training session before you make your decision. Look for two-way communication between the trainer and the boxer, instruction that is clear, direct, patient, and consistent without a demeaning, reprimanding, or criticizing manner. A good trainer will bring out the best in you and place you on a schedule specific to your skill level and needs. He should identify your strengths and weaknesses and recognize that everyone progresses at his or her own rate.

Be honest with your trainer about your fitness level. This is especially important before each training session. Sparring is part of the training that requires good conditioning because of the possibility of getting hurt. If you have not been training or are not up to your normal physical condition, the trainer may delay the sparring session or adjust the intensity according to your physical condition.

The trainer will want to see your abilities and conditioning level before a decision will be made if you are ready to spar. When the boxer feels ready and the trainer agrees then a sparring match is set. Do not even think about sparring unless you have the conditioning. The trainer will pick sparring partners and oversee the sparring sessions. He or she will also ensure that the sparring is controlled and that an experienced boxer helps a less experienced boxer

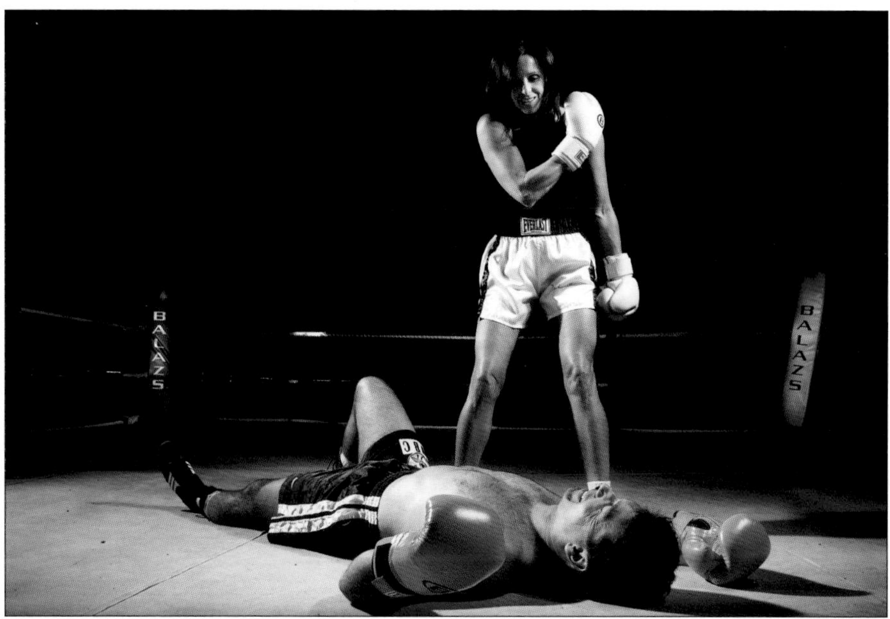

rather than taking advantage of the inexperience. Boxing training and sparring should be fun, not a struggle to keep from getting hurt.

Until the Last Bell

Take inventory of your life, and remember that the path you follow today is an investment in every day that is still to come. Whatever fitness activities you choose to be involved in, take pride in your performance, work the basics, and enjoy the journey. Give yourself time to adapt, and grow and make fitness a long-term, lifetime commitment, and a regular part of your everyday life. Make fitness your personal journey.

Acknowledgments

Special thanks to:

The Great Julio Cesar Chavez, Jose Sulaiman and Mauricio Sulaiman of the World Boxing Council.
Jill Diamond, WBC female championship committee.
Jeanie Kahnke of the Muhammad Ali Center.
Troy Moth, Jeff Julian, Ivan Krolo.
Balazs Boxing—John Kim of Jump USA, and Marty Winkler and Louis Garcia of Free-Style Jump Roping.
John Melich of Champion Boxing Club.
John Poirier and everyone at the Gym.

About the Authors

Andy Dumas is one of Canada's leading fitness experts. Born into a boxing background, he had the fortune of growing up in an environment that promoted physical activity and boxing training. At a young age, Andy started hitting the heavy bag, working on his rhythm on the speed bag, jumping rope, and fighting in the ring.

As a Canadian boxing coach and a certified fitness consultant, he understands the long hours of training, the commitment to the sport, and the intense mental focus required by the very best-conditioned athlete.

As a sought after fitness presenter, Andy has been featured at major fitness conferences, various educational facilities, and is the host and producer of T.V. fitness/sports shows. His projects include the "The One-Two Punch," "i-box," "Roadwork for Boxers," and "Training Camp."

Andy promotes cross-training and believes fitness is essential to good living. He lives, writes, teaches, and works out in Oakville, Ontario, Canada.

Jamie Dumas is a firm believer that fitness is for absolutely everyone. With an Honors Bachelor of Science Degree in Human Kinetics from the University of Waterloo, Ontario, Canada, she has extensive experience in the fitness industry, managing fitness centers, providing personal training, and motivating the inactive. She is a trainer of fitness instructors and develops and implements a variety of programs and workshops for fitness clubs. She divides her time between developing new fitness programs and exploring avenues to share her passion in health and fitness with the community.

Andy and Jamie are the resident fitness experts on the Canadian T.V. show Real Life. This half-hour show explores and discusses a variety of interests, activities, and hobbies, placing a positive spin on real life. Andy also runs the fitness website www.andydumas.ca.

Index

C

Notes

NOTES

Notes

NOTES